ANTI-INFLAMMATORY DIET
FOR BEGINNERS

THE PAIN-FREE ANTI-INFLAMMATORY COOKBOOK FOR BEGINNERS:

Detox Your Body & Boost Immunity with Easy & Tasty Natural Recipes

Includes Advice from over 3700 Interviews
(12-Week Meal Plan Included)

FAN CLUB KITCHEN is a young and independent publishing house that collaborates with expert chefs and nutritionists to create guides and cookbooks for various types of diets.

What sets THE FAN CLUB KITCHEN's books apart is the fact that all of them are created with the help of fans, readers, and followers who actively participate in their creation alongside nutrition experts. Thousands of interviews are conducted prior to the creation of a new book, giving voice to ordinary people and bringing their needs, curiosities, and problems to the forefront.

Our goal is to unite the experiences of dieticians, qualified doctors, and chefs with those of ordinary people, bringing together their advice on nutrition and cooking tips in a single book.

By putting the spotlight on everyday individuals, we hope to create a brand that resonates with a wide audience and meets their specific needs in a personal and engaging way. We're proud to be different from traditional publishers and believe that our unique approach to cookbook creation will help us stand out and create a loyal fan base.

At **FAN CLUB KITCHEN**, we believe that cookbooks should be more than just recipes. That's why we're excited to introduce our latest book on the anti-inflammatory diet, a project that has been months in the making.

Our dedicated team has conducted over 3,000 interviews to gather the doubts and fears of people who are embarking on the journey of an anti-inflammatory diet.

Through these interviews, we've discovered the numerous needs that people have, from understanding the right foods to bring to the table to figuring out why certain foods trigger inflammation in our bodies.

We've also heard from busy individuals who are looking for ways to start a healthy diet without breaking the bank or spending too much time in the kitchen.

With all of this feedback, we've created the perfect guide for those looking to adopt an anti-inflammatory diet, even if they're starting from scratch.

Our collaborator, Marlissa, has brought her expertise and experience to the project, making this book an essential resource for anyone looking to improve their health through nutrition.

We believe that everyone deserves access to healthy eating, and we're proud to offer our latest book as a valuable resource for anyone looking to live their best life.

Marlissa, our Holistic Health Coach! Marlissa understands firsthand the challenges of dealing with chronic illness and struggling to find a path to wellness. In 2020, she found herself bedridden most days with over 40 chronic illness symptoms, struggling to make it through the day without excessive stimulants, and drowning in debt from all the broken promises of courses, supplements, and detox kits. She knew she couldn't continue living this way.

After years of setbacks and challenges, Marlissa had a breakthrough and discovered how to detox her way out of disease, pain, and inflammation. She created a system that allows individuals like us, who are driven, high-achieving, and committed, to manifest dynamic health through an anti-inflammatory, alkaline diet.

An anti-inflammatory diet is about eating more real, whole foods and less processed foods, with the goal of reducing inflammation in the body. Chronic inflammation is linked to a host of diseases and conditions, so an anti-inflammatory diet is an overall, good diet for most people to consider. With Marlissa's guidance, you can incorporate foods that help you fight disease and not feed disease.

Marlissa's proven system has allowed her to heal from all 40 of her chronic illness symptoms, start an online holistic healing mentorship business that changes lives, and work with clients from around the globe who want better gut and overall health. She structures her healing programs based on her own journey that is proven to work seamlessly every time, working with clients on a specific nutritional plan based on healing the body through food from an anti-inflammatory diet.

In this book, Marlissa collaborates with us to create a guide that outlines the steps you can take to start a holistic lifestyle without spending too much money. The guide explains how to wake up with more energy, get out of bed with greater vitality, and most importantly, fight chronic pain.

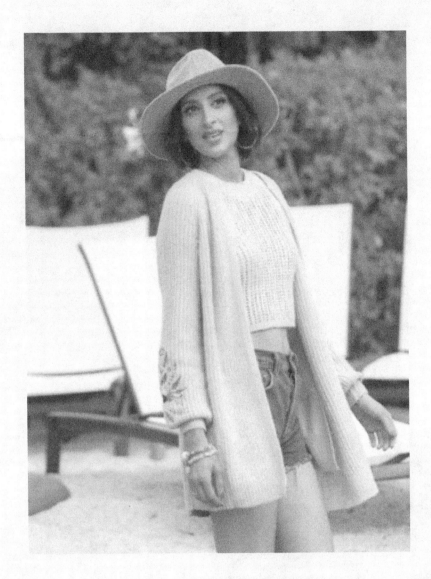

Are you ready to revolutionize your diet and achieve optimal health and vitality?

At the end of this book, you will discover an exclusive gift for our readers. You will have the opportunity to get a plan perfectly tailored to your needs for changing your diet, thanks to the expertise of our Holistic Health Coach, Marlissa.

And as if that wasn't enough, in addition, you will discover an incredible bonus tagged Fan Club kitchen, but we won't reveal further you will find out everything on the last page of this book.

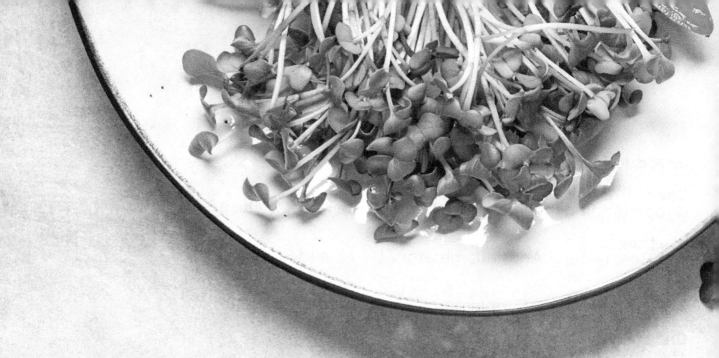

Introduction

Chronic inflammation is a major cause of many diseases. Although drugs are an option, diet changes are frequently more effective in reducing inflammation. This book will show you how to get started with a simple anti-inflammatory diet plan that is simple to follow and free!

If your joints, muscles, or tendons hurt when you move, anti-inflammatory medication is the solution. While there are medications that can help reduce inflammation, eating anti-inflammatory foods can help improve quality of life. The Anti-Inflammatory Diet can help with this. The anti-inflammatory diet is widely regarded as the healthiest diet available to people. It encourages people to eat foods that reduce inflammation in the body.

Following the Anti-Inflammatory Diet, I created this book because I believe that eating the right foods can help reduce chronic inflammation. Wouldn't you think life is better if you could improve your health with food? Moreover, this book also contains simple and easy-to-follow recipes for everyone. While I have included everything you need to know about the Anti-Inflammatory Diet in this book, I want to ensure that all readers understand the concepts of this specific diet.

However, while the Anti-Inflammatory Diet may help improve the condition of people suffering from chronic inflammation, it does not completely heal individuals and only reduces flare-ups. However, if you want to improve your condition, you should not only rely on this diet, but also exercise, live a healthy lifestyle, take your medication, and consult with your medical practitioner.

This book will teach you about an anti-inflammatory diet, what it is, and why you should consider it instead of medication. This cookbook will get you started on the path to discovering the diet that gives you the most life, energy, and comfort.

This cookbook is for anyone who wants to experiment with their diet and improve the quality of their lifestyle without sacrificing flavor. Anti-inflammatory cooking may be more effective than traditional medicine in treating autoimmune diseases such as rheumatoid arthritis, lupus, and others! This is also a book for people who want to eat healthier but don't have time to spend hours in the kitchen every day. The recipes below are some of our family's favorites that we believe should be on any healthy-eating menu plan. Let's get started.

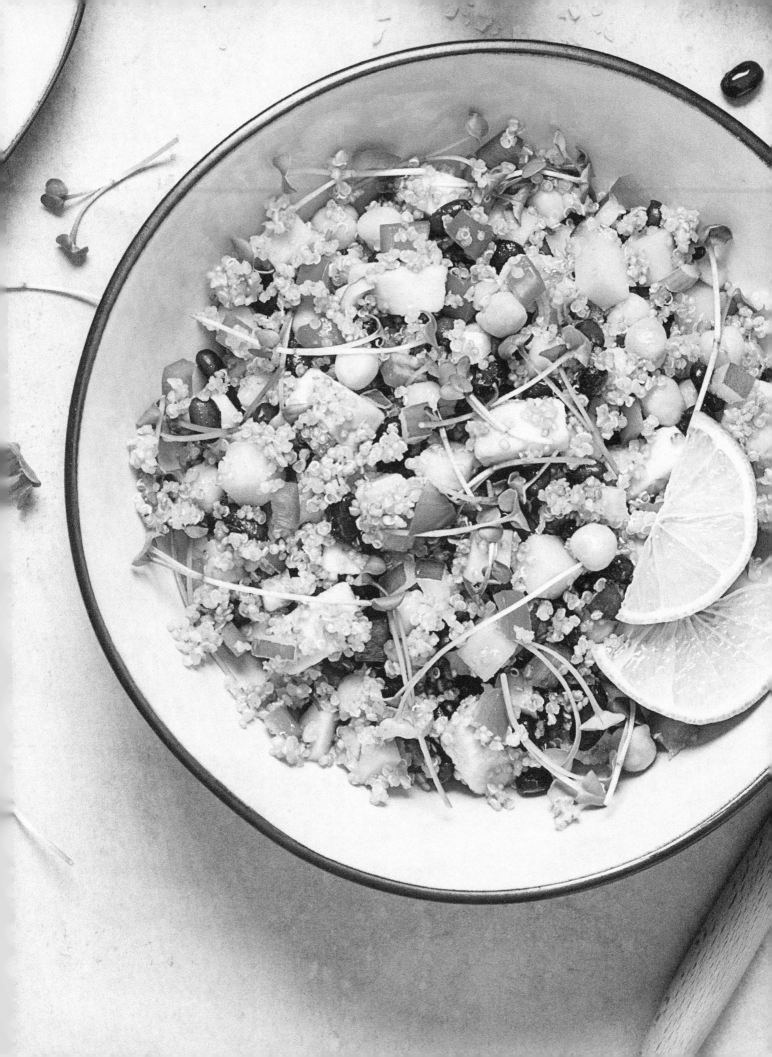

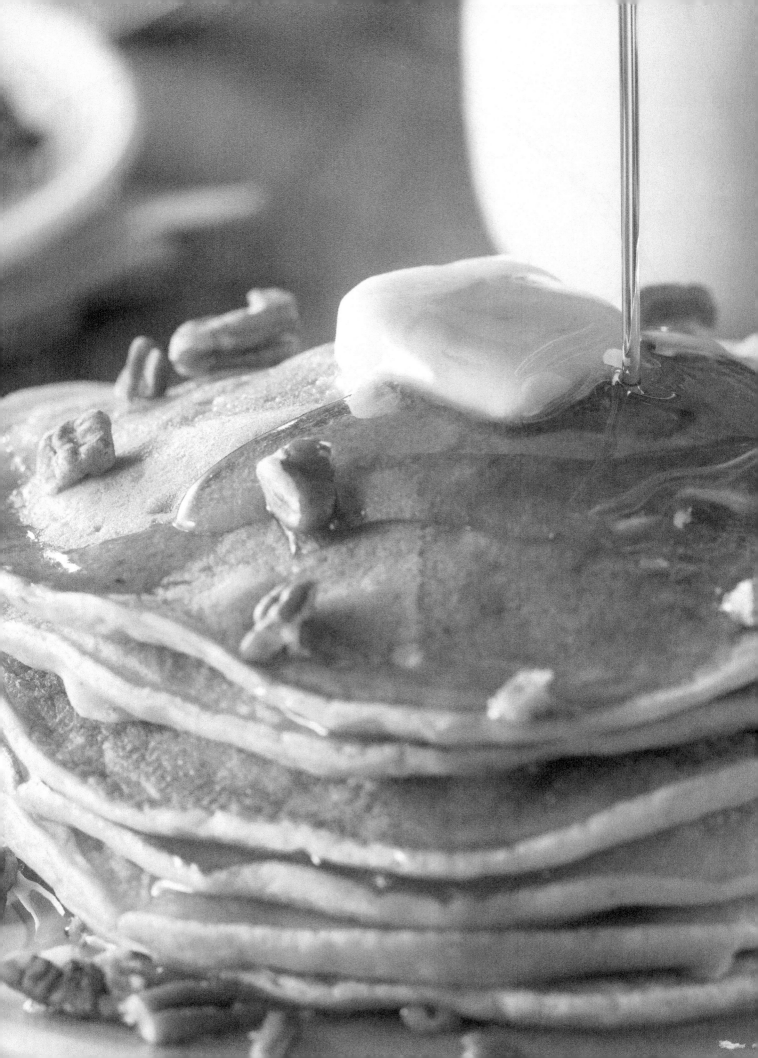

Chapter 1:

Understanding Inflammation:

The Importance of Diet

What is Inflammation?

Inflammation is a completely natural process that your body uses to fight off anything harmful. If you scrape your knee, for example, your immune system responds by healing the wound. Acute inflammation is a part of this process because it stimulates the production of white blood cells, immune cells, and other substances that promote healing and aid in infection resistance.

Inflammation is produced in response to injury, illness, or infection to protect and heal tissues, cells, and organs. While inflammation is initially beneficial to the body, it can become a problem if it becomes chronic. Chronic inflammation is the root cause of allergies, type II diabetes, irritable bowel syndrome (IBS), heart disease, and cancer.

There are two types of inflammation: acute and chronic. Acute inflammation is caused by an injury, such as a scratch or cut, sprained ankle, or sore throat. In this case, the immune system only responds to the injured area. The inflammation is only present for as long as the damage is repaired. It would dilate the red blood vessels, increasing blood flow. White blood cells would multiply in the affected area, assisting in the body's healing. Redness, swelling, pain, a warm sensation, or fever are all symptoms of acute inflammation.

During acute inflammation, the damaged tissue releases a chemical called cytokines. Cytokines signal our bodies to send more white blood cells and nutrients to help with healing. Prostaglandins, a hormone-like substance, cause pain and fever while also forming blood clots that help with tissue repair. As the body heals, the inflammation diminishes until it is no longer required.

While acute inflammation can help the body heal itself, chronic inflammation can cause more harm than good. Chronic inflammation is usually found at low levels all over the body. The term "suicide" refers to the act of killing someone. It also refers to the act of committing suicide.

Chronic inflammation can be caused by anything the body perceives as a threat, no matter how real it is. This inflammation still causes white blood cells to respond, but because nothing needs their attention to heal, they may start attacking healthy cells, tissues, and organs. While researchers are still trying to figure out how chronic inflammation works, they do know that it increases the likelihood of the development of many diseases.

Chronic inflammation causes diseases such as type II diabetes, Alzheimer's disease, obesity, and even depression. Chronic inflammation, if left untreated, can cause tissue or organ damage over time.

This is a temporary condition characterized by swelling, redness, pain, and some heat radiating from the injured area.

Chronic inflammation, on the other hand, is not always visible and occurs primarily within the body. Unhealed infections, obesity, autoimmune disease, and prolonged exposure to environmental toxins such as cigarette smoke can all cause acute inflammation to progress to chronic inflammation. Diabetes, fatty liver disease, Alzheimer's disease, heart disease, and a variety of other ailments can result from this.

As you can see, acute inflammation is nothing to worry about, but it is when this natural response is not resolved and turns into chronic inflammation when there's cause for concern.

These are some symptoms you can look out for that may indicate that you are experiencing chronic inflammation.

- High blood pressure
- Insulin resistance
- Memory loss
- Depression
- Joint pain
- Stiffness
- Bloating and gas
- Constipation
- Lack of energy
- Weight gain
- Inability to lose weight
- High level of bad cholesterol (LDL) and low level of good cholesterol (HDL)
- Mouth sores
- Recurrent rashes

A variety of factors can trigger an inflammatory response in the body, including stress, lack of sleep, and certain medications. Other causes may include viruses or bacteria which invade your system, causing infectious diseases which lead to inflammation to fight it off after being attacked by these harmful agents. Unhealthy eating is one of the most common reasons for developing high levels of chronic inflammation because food directly impacts how our bodies function.

When it comes to inflammation, diet is one of the most important factors that affect how your body reacts. The food we eat every day, such as junk food and processed treats, contributes to chronic inflammation in our bodies because they lack anti-inflammatory elements, not providing enough nutrients to keep us healthy.

The best way to combat inflammation is through diet rather than drugs because drugs only suppress symptoms while never addressing the root problem caused by improper eating habits. When it comes to inflammation, food directly impacts how our bodies function, which is why we need anti-inflammatory foods that reduce the effects of chronic inflammation to maintain optimum health. These foods include omega-rich fish such as wild salmon, avocado oil, green leafy vegetables like kale or spinach, almonds and walnuts for their healthy fats content, among other superfoods rich in nutrients that are known for fighting off infections effectively without causing any side effects if taken properly.

Anti-inflammation diet helps the human body by reducing the pain and inflammation caused by inflammatory issues. It reduces symptoms of autoimmune diseases such as arthritis, lupus, psoriasis, ulcerative colitis, etc., by helping the body heal itself.

Importance of Anti-Inflammatory Diet

The anti-inflammatory diet focuses on lowering inflammatory markers in the body. This can be accomplished by consuming anti-inflammatory foods such as fruits, fish, vegetables, and healthy fats. Furthermore, this diet encourages people to eat moderate amounts of red meat, nuts, and wine. However, there are other factors to consider when following this diet in addition to eating healthy foods. The emphasis is on a well-balanced diet rich in vegetables and fruits. These low-calorie foods aid digestion and weight management and reduce inflammation, thereby preventing cellular damage. Brightly colored fruits and vegetables are especially healthy because they contain more phytochemicals, which are plant compounds that have been shown to reduce inflammation.

Refined grains are preferred over whole grains. Unrefined grains high in fiber, antioxidants, and other nutrients that are beneficial to your health include oats, quinoa, barley, chia, and sorghum. Whole grains help the body's immune system by providing valuable nourishment to beneficial gut bacteria. Other high-fiber foods, such as beans, and fermented foods, such as kefir, kimchi, and pickles, help to balance gut bacteria while also fighting inflammation and disease.

When it comes to fats, the anti-inflammatory diet recommends choosing plant-based options such as olive oil over trans fats and saturated fats found in animal products. Olive oil has been shown to have numerous health benefits.

It is also strongly advised to increase your intake of omega-3 fats. This healthy fat reduces inflammation directly. Fish and walnuts are high in omega-3 fatty acids. Most other nuts and seeds contain healthy fats, protein, and other important micronutrients that can help boost your immune system.

Red meat consumption is restricted to the anti-inflammatory diet because it contains high levels of undesirable fats, sodium, antibiotics, and hormones, all of which increase inflammation. Cooking methods such as grilling should be avoided when eating red meat because the blackened parts of the meat can cause inflammation. Fish and poultry are better choices for animal protein in general.

Because of their high antioxidant content, green tea and red wine are two popular anti-inflammatory beverages. You are also permitted to consume coffee. And, of course, you can't go wrong with drinking water.

Fresh fruits and vegetables must be included in an anti-inflammatory lunch. Antioxidants are abundant in plant-based diets. Certain foods, on the other hand, may cause the body to produce radicals. One example is food cooked in oil that has been heated repeatedly.

Dietary antioxidants, or substances found in food, assist the body in eliminating free radicals. Body processes such as metabolism generate free radicals, which are then released into the environment. However, external factors, such as stress or cigarette use, can increase the body's level of free radicals.

Although eating antioxidants is beneficial, the body naturally produces antioxidants that aid in the removal of this toxic comb.

When leading an anti-inflammatory lifestyle, foods strong in antioxidants are recommended over those that increase levels of free radicals.

Omega-3 fatty acids, which are included in oily fish like salmon and tuna, may help reduce the body's synthesis of inflammatory mediators. The Arthritis Foundation claims that fiber could have a comparable effect.

Lifestyle Changes

The effect your lifestyle has on your health is undeniable.

Individuals who experience chronic psychological stress are more likely to develop heart disease, depression, and anxiety. These people's bodies are also more likely to lose their ability to defend themselves and regulate their inflammatory processes. Relaxing the nervous system has been shown to have far-reaching effects in alleviating, managing, and reducing the far-reaching and harmful effects of stress-induced chronic inflammation on the immune system and the body as a whole. Individuals who practice stress management techniques have higher levels of anti-inflammatory gene expression and lower levels of inflammatory gene expression. These effects can be obtained by simply listening to a 20-minute guided meditation a few times per week, practicing deep-breathing exercises, or incorporating yoga and Tai Chi into your weekly routine.

Stress management is critical for controlling inflammation levels in the body. Although stress is a natural part of life, if it is not addressed, a person's body will lose the ability to respond to excessive cortisol (stress hormone) release in a healthy manner, resulting in increased inflammation.

Sleep is another important factor in maintaining your health because it allows your body to recover and repair any damage. You are more likely to develop chronic inflammation and other health issues, such as type 2 diabetes and weight gain, if you do not get enough restful sleep.

Exercising for 30 minutes five days a week at a moderate intensity or for 1 hour and 15 minutes at a high intensity significantly reduces inflammation while also contributing to overall well-being. Physical activity also helps with stress management, so you'll be killing two birds with one stone! Exercise on a regular basis is extremely beneficial to your sympathetic nervous system. 20-minute exercise sessions have been shown in studies to benefit your immune system and thus reduce inflammation measurably. This advantage stems from the fact that the energy expenditure associated with exercise has been clinically proven to reduce the body's production of a variety of pro-inflammatory cytokines and molecules.

Regular exercise helps to control weight, strengthen the heart, bones, and muscles, and lower the risk of cardiovascular disease, in addition to strengthening the immune system. So, whether you go for a 20-minute walk or spend 2 hours at the gym, getting some kind of physical activity, even if it's just a 20-minute walk, will help keep that inflammation under control.

Stop Smoking and excessive alcohol. Smoking and excessive alcohol consumption also dramatically increase inflammation in the body — for obvious reasons — and should be ceased for your well-being.

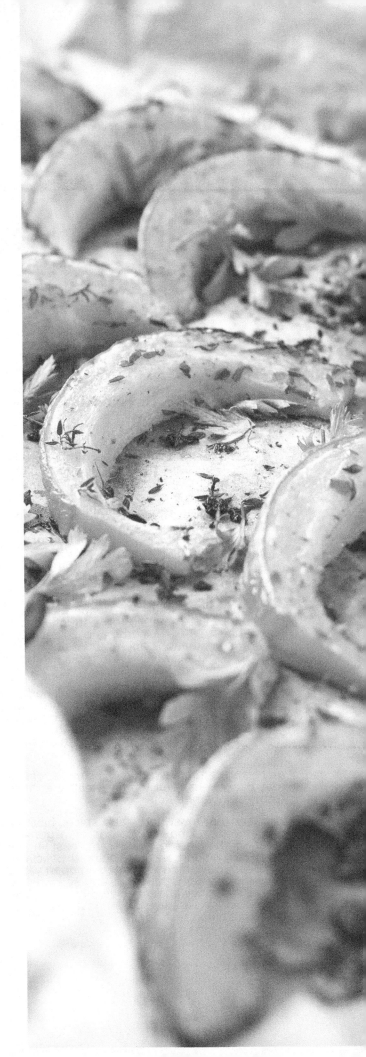

11

Chapter 2:

The Best Natural Anti-Inflammatory Herbs and Spices

What Role Do Herbs and Spices Play In Reducing Inflammation?

Herbs and spices have long been used to reduce inflammation. Spices like turmeric have been used for thousands of years to treat inflammation and inflammation-related conditions like arthritis.

Various spices and herbs have recently been studied in experimental settings and discovered to be effective in reducing inflammation or symptoms of inflammation-based diseases. These effects can be significant and more potent than some non-steroid anti-inflammatory drugs.

The gist is that some herbs and spices contain chemicals that either reduce or increase the body's pro-inflammatory or anti-inflammatory substances. Different herbs and spices contain varying combinations and amounts of such beneficial chemicals, which act to reduce inflammation in various ways.

However, as one might expect, not all herbs and spices are equally beneficial. Herbs and spices, like other plants and plant products, contain chemicals that are good for us, some that are bad for us, some that are a mix of both, and some that don't seem to do much for us at all.

Anise and cardamom are two examples of spices that may be harmful to your health, at least in terms of inflammation.

The fact that most herbs and spices have been used for thousands of years is an argument in favor of their being healthy, at least in doses used for cooking and seasoning. I believe that the best you can do is to keep an open yet critical mind, try something out, and see whether it makes a positive impact on your health, whether by keeping a close eye on your symptoms, or by getting a blood test done.

Anti-Inflammatory Herbs and Spices

The following list of herbs and spices is based on my own research. For all of the herbs and spices on the list, I believe that there is adequate evidence that they actually do help in reducing inflammation. All the listed herbs and spices have been studied in vitro (meaning isolated cells outside of living organisms) as well as in animals using concentrated amounts. Also, most of these herbs and spices have been studied using extracts or concentrated doses in human subjects with good effect. Finally, several (turmeric, ginger, cloves, and rosemary) have also been shown to help reduce inflammation when used only as a culinary spice rather than as an extract in a capsule.

Turmeric

Turmeric is most commonly available as a dried, ground form of the root, though fresh root may be available as well. It has long been used for dyeing, as a key ingredient in curries, and to color mustards. It has also been used in traditional Indian medicine to treat a variety of ailments.

Turmeric is an important component of curry seasoning. It can also be used to flavor and color rice, season meat, and in salads and salad dressings. It's ultimately up to you, and turmeric is a versatile spice that can be used in a variety of ways.

Black Pepper

Black pepper is such a versatile spice that it can be used in almost any dish. You can add it during any step of the cooking process. To preserve the piperine, the active ingredient that provides spiciness and aids in turmeric absorption, wait until the end because heat will decompose piperine to some extent.

Ginger

Zingiber officinale, or ginger, is a flowering perennial plant. Ginger was originally from China, but India is now the largest producer.

Ginger's anti-inflammatory properties have been studied both in vitro and in human subjects. In both types of studies, it was found to have a significant effect on reducing pro-inflammatory substances. In addition, ginger is used to relieve pain and soothe upset stomachs.

Ginger is commonly used as a spice in many Asian cuisines to flavor both meats and vegetables. It is more commonly used in the West to flavor cookies and sweets, and it is also used as a spice in tea and coffee. When cooking with ginger, a little goes a long way, so start slowly if you're not sure how much you'll need.

Cloves

Cloves are derived from the Syzygium aromaticum, a large evergreen tree native to Indonesia but now cultivated throughout the Indian Ocean. This spice is made from the aromatic flower buds of the tree, which are picked and dried until hard and brown. Cloves are typically sold as whole flower buds, though ground clove powder is also available.

Cloves have been shown to reduce inflammation in both in vitro and human trials. Importantly, the reduced inflammation was noticeable even at normal cooking amounts. Cloves appear to help reduce the symptoms of rheumatoid arthritis as well. Furthermore, cloves have long been used for pain relief, particularly in dentistry.

Basil

Different types of basil contain eugenol, the same compound found in cloves and responsible for much of their medicinal value. Holy basil, which contains more eugenol than sweet basil, has been extensively studied for its medicinal properties, and it has been discovered to have anti-inflammatory, pain-killing, and anti-microbial properties.

While sweet basil contains less eugenol, it still appears to have anti-inflammatory properties, and I use it in cooking all the time because I love the aroma. It goes well with tomatoes and is a popular ingredient in Italian cuisine. It can be used to season sauces and salads, and is a key ingredient in pesto. At the end of cooking, add fresh basil leaves, whole or chopped, to preserve their flavor and aroma as well as the compounds that provide anti-inflammatory benefits.

Sage

Sage, also known as Salvia officinalis, is a Mediterranean perennial shrub.

Sage contains rosmarinic acid, which has anti-inflammatory and antioxidant properties (also found in rosemary). The beneficial effects of sage have been discovered in both in vitro and human studies, using both extracts and just fresh herbs.

Sage is especially useful for seasoning fatty meats and stuffings when cooking. It's a powerful herb that can easily overpower a dish. When cooking, use it sparingly.

Rosemary

Rosemary, like the other herbs on this list, has antioxidant and anti-inflammatory properties. In cooking, rosemary has been shown in studies to be effective in reducing inflammation. Furthermore, rosemary appears to reduce anxiety and may aid in memory enhancement.

Rosemary is commonly used to season meats, fish, and stuffing. It can also be used to flavor pasta sauces, oven-baked potatoes, and oils or butter. As with other herbs, rosemary can be used to make tea.

Cinnamon

Cinnamon is used to flavor a variety of desserts, pastries, and chocolate. It's commonly used in hot drinks like coffee and tea. It is also used to flavor meat, such as chicken or lamb, in several Middle Eastern cuisines.

Cinnamon is unlikely to cause significant side effects when used in normal cooking quantities. However, there are some concerns if you plan to consume larger amounts of cinnamon. Cinnamomum cassia, the most common commercially available form of cinnamon, contains coumarin, a substance that, in high doses, can cause liver and kidney damage.

Oregano

Oregano is popular in Italian cuisine and is particularly common on pizzas. It is also used for seasoning meats, fish, and fried or grilled vegetables.

As for concentrated or supplemental versions of oregano, there is an essential oil that is extracted from oregano leaves, and it is used in aromatherapy. It's also possible to get gelcaps containing oregano oil for internal use. Also, while many people ingest oregano oil successfully, there appear to be equally as many cases of strongly upset stomachs and other intestinal problems.

Chapter 3:

Anti-Inflammatory Supplements That Actually Work

Natural Anti-Inflammatory Supplement Options

Take caution when deciding whether or not to incorporate supplements into your diet, as supplements are largely unregulated and can cause side effects such as nose bleeds, nausea, loose stools, gas, and bad breath. Check with your regular healthcare provider before incorporating any supplements into your diet, especially if you are dealing with any specific medical issues or are currently taking any medications.

While supplements can help you develop and maintain a healthy lifestyle, they should not be used as a substitute for professional healthcare or to replace a healthy diet. It's also worth noting that many of the nutrients listed above can be obtained naturally by eating specific types of whole foods. The benefit of supplements, on the other hand, is that the body receives a much higher dose of those nutrients than it would by simply eating whole foods.

Several popular brands of supplements, particularly multivitamins that are widely available in drug stores, contain a vitamin that the body cannot readily utilize; they are essentially placebos. As a result, it is critical to conduct research on the type and brand of any supplement being considered and ensure that the research is coming from a reliable source.

Given the numerous health benefits associated with anti-oxidants, it may be tempting to incorporate some anti-oxidant supplements into your daily diet routine. When deciding whether to take antioxidant supplements, keep in mind that the majority of clinical studies on antioxidant supplements have found that they do not provide any significant health benefits, so your best bet is to get your antioxidants the old-fashioned way.

Omega-3 fatty acids are essential in any diet, but they are especially beneficial in the treatment of inflammatory disorders. One of the primary causes of inflammation is an excess of omega-6 fatty acids, which are commonly found in proces-

sed foods. However, consuming more omega-3 can offset the negative effects of omega-6.

By reducing inflammation in the body, omega-3 reduces the risk of cancer and asthma. Fish oil capsules, which are available in most vitamin aisles, can provide your daily dose of omega-3.

Vitamin D3 is a hormone-like vitamin that our skin can produce if exposed to sunlight for an extended period of time each day. However, because most modern people live indoors and sunscreens are widely used to protect against skin cancer, a large proportion of the population is dangerously low or deficient in vitamin D. Inflammatory skin conditions, asthma, arthritis, diabetes, and cancer are just a few of the many health risks associated with low vitamin D levels.

Vitamins C and E are antioxidant vitamins that, while old school, i.e., boring, are still extremely important in our fad-driven society. Antihistamine properties of vitamin C can help to reduce allergic inflammation. Vitamin E may inhibit the activation of mast cells, which are also involved in allergic reactions.

Curcumin is a natural anti-inflammatory ingredient found in the popular Indian spice turmeric, and it is also available as a supplement. Turmeric has traditionally been used in Ayurvedic medicine to treat a variety of conditions, including arthritis and asthma. Ingesting curcumin relieves joint pain caused by inflammatory diseases. Curcumin, in more absorbable forms, may help slow the progression of Alzheimer's disease, which causes irreversible damage to brain cells that control memory.

Magnesium is a mineral that helps to keep blood pressure stable and bones strong. Magnesium aids in the prevention of arterial wall inflammation. Increased magnesium consumption can lower the indicator TNF, which regulates the immune system but can also cause inflammation. One reason magnesium has been linked to a lower risk of heart disease may be due to its anti-inflammatory properties.

Zinc is a metal that aids in the suppression of the

body's immune response.

Ginger has been used for thousands of years in Ayurvedic medicine to treat arthritis. Gingerols are anti-inflammatory compounds found in this root. Ginger protects the body's lipids from free radical damage. It also inhibits the production of inflammatory compounds in the joints. When patients consume ginger on a daily basis, their joint pain and swelling can be significantly reduced.

Resveratrol is a plant extract derived from peanuts as well as fruits such as grapes. It is frequently used to treat inflammatory bowel disease symptoms. Several studies have found a link between resveratrol consumption and suppression of the inflammatory protein TNF-alpha. Resveratrol has also been linked to longevity in fruit flies and may help humans live longer lives.

Alpha-lipoic acid is well-known as an antioxidant, but it is also an effective anti-inflammatory agent. It guards against nerve damage caused by low oxygen levels, free radicals, high blood sugar levels, and even aging. Alpha-lipoic acid can provide drug-free pain relief to diabetics with diabetic neuropathy. It may benefit bone health by reducing inflammation-induced bone loss. Alpha-lipoic acid may also alleviate inflammatory symptoms associated with multiple sclerosis.

Quercetin is an antioxidant and anti-inflammatory plant pigment. It is especially beneficial in the treatment of heart and blood vessel problems. Its anti-inflammatory properties can help with fibromyalgia pain. Because quercetin can reduce oxidative damage to the brain, certain highly bioavailable forms of this plant pigment may help protect against neurodegenerative diseases such as Alzheimer's and Parkinson's.

Milk thistle is a flowering herb native to the Mediterranean that is best known for promoting liver health. The active ingredient in milk thistle, silymarin, heals liver cell damage. The herb reduces liver inflammation and aids in the recovery from hepatitis. Milk thistle is also used to treat gallbladder inflammation.

Vitamin K2 is a type of Vitamin K produced primarily by bacteria in the stomach. Vitamin K1 is also beneficial because it aids in blood clotting. In the body, K1 can be converted to K2. However, some forms of Vitamin K2 have anti-inflammatory properties, and it is best to absorb it directly to reap the most benefit. By reducing inflammation, vitamin K2 can protect against cardiovascular disease and osteoporosis. If you must take anticoagulant medication such as Coumadin or Warfarin, consult your doctor before using any vitamin K products.

Antibiotics or yeast infections can cause an overgrowth of bad bacteria, resulting in poor immune system function throughout your body. When your intestinal bacteria are out of balance, inflammation can occur. According to some research, certain multi-strain probiotics may reduce the severity of inflammatory bowel disease and Crohn's disease in people with those difficult chronic gastrointestinal inflammatory conditions.

Many of these vitamins and herbs are beneficial additions to your daily vitamin regimen and have few to no side effects. They are widely available in supermarkets, drug stores, and health food stores.

If you are suffering from an inflammatory condition but are concerned about complications from NSAIDs, you may want to supplement your diet with anti-inflammatory herbs and minerals. Then work with your own healthcare provider to see if it is possible for you to taper and perhaps stop the drugs over time.

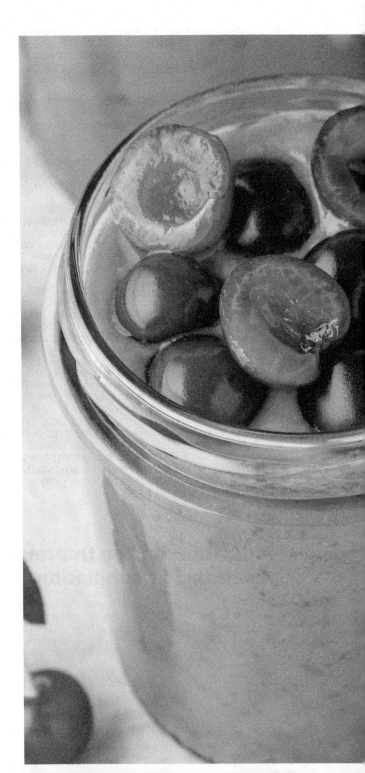

15

Chapter 4:

The Best Natural Alternatives to NSAIDs

Inflammation control is critical to your overall health and well-being. The method you use to control it can either be extremely effective or cause even more health problems than the amount you started with.

A common misconception about "treating" chronic inflammation is that inflammation is the primary problem. This misconception frequently leads to people attempting to reduce inflammation without addressing the underlying cause. Chronic inflammation, rather than being the ongoing problem itself, is the body's ongoing attempt to address some ongoing problem.

When only reducing inflammation is attempted, the body's natural healing process is disrupted, halted, and/or otherwise interfered with. Continued disruption of the healing process will weaken the body's natural defenses, exacerbating the issues that caused the inflammation in the first place.

The point is that while controlling inflammation is critical to maintaining your health and well-being, it is also critical to do so by focusing on the cause of the inflammation rather than the inflammation itself.

Keep in mind that your body is not stupid, and it is constantly working to keep you alive. If your body is triggering your immune system to the point of causing chronic inflammation, it is because your body is attempting to deal with an ongoing stimulus that it perceives as a threat. Make the mistake of believing that your body is inflamed despite itself. Your body initiates the inflammatory process for a reason, and constantly stopping or disrupting that process prevents the body from defending itself.

Medication for the treatment of Chronic Inflammation

While treating chronic inflammation with medication can be beneficial in some cases. Chronic inflammation should always be treated with caution and under the supervision of a healthcare professional. Remember that no medication has a single effect; all medications have side effects. This means that when you take one medication to treat one symptom, it comes at the expense of another. In fact, the side effects of one medication may necessitate the prescription of a different medication to treat that side effect. The circle continues indefinitely.

Because all medications have side effects, they are ineffective in establishing and maintaining long-term health.

The following medications are commonly used to treat chronic inflammation:

Steroids

Corticosteroids, such as cortisone and prednisone, are steroid hormones that are commonly used to reduce systemic inflammation in conditions such as allergic asthma and arthritis. Corticosteroids accomplish this by suppressing many of the pathways in the body that contribute to the inflammatory process. When the immune system begins to target the body's own healthy tissue, suppressing the immune system's response to allergens in this way can be beneficial. On the other hand, long-term use of steroids has been linked to a slew of health issues. Hypertension, osteoporosis, vision problems, weight gain, and fluid retention are among the health issues. "Glucocorticoids" are another form of steroid that is generally used to treat inflammatory conditions such as asthma, inflammatory arthritis, sarcoidosis, and systemic lupus.

Nonsteroidal Anti-Inflammatory Medication (NSAIDs)

As the name implies, NSAIDs reduce inflammation but are unrelated to steroids and are generally safe for occasional use if taken as directed. There are three commonly used OTC NSAIDs. Ibuprofen, the active ingredient in Advil and Motrin, is the first. The active ingredient in Aleve is naproxen, the second most common NSAID. Aspirin is the third most commonly used over-the-counter NSAID.

NSAIDs work by decreasing the body's production of prostaglandins. "Prostaglandins" are physiological chemicals known as "eicosanoids" that are similar to hormones and play a significant role in the inflammatory process. Prostaglandins cause increased blood flow, chemotaxis, and tissue and organ dysfunction as a result. As a result, prostaglandins have a wide range of hormone-like effects on the body, which can manifest as fever, pain, and/or inflammation. As a result of limiting prostaglandin production, NSAIDs reduce fever, pain, and inflammation. It is important to note that acetaminophen (Tylenol), while commonly used to treat pain, has no effect on inflammation.

However, because prostaglandins protect the lining of the stomach and intestines, long-term use of NSAIDs can result in stomach and intestine ulcers, peptic ulcer disease, and an increased risk of bleeding. This disruption in the gut's microbiome can, ironically, cause more inflammation in the intestinal walls (commonly known as "leaky gut"), resulting in the release of toxins and, as a result, chronic inflammation throughout the body. Long-term NSAID use can also result in progressive kidney damage, sudden kidney failure, and/or chronic interstitial nephritis, a type of chronic kidney disease.

Because of the risky long-term effects of NSAIDs, they should only be used under the supervision of a healthcare professional if you have heart, liver, or kidney disease, hypertension, are over the age of 65, or take diuretics. If you do decide to use over-the-counter NSAIDs, it is best to limit your use to no more than 10 days for pain relief and no more than three days for fever reduction. If you have pain or a fever for more than 10 days or 3 days, respectively, you should see a doctor.

Metformin

Metformin is a medication that is commonly used to treat type 2 diabetes and chronic low-grade inflammation. Metformin has been shown to reduce inflammation by inhibiting the body's production of pro-inflammatory cytokines, such as macrophages, which normally activate the immune system. The term "macrophage" refers to a type of white blood cell that is responsible for the detection, phagocytosis (or "ingestion"), and eventual destruction of harmful organisms such as allergens, toxins, and pathogens. When the body's production of the immune cells that cause inflammation is inhibited, the inflammation is also inhibited.

Metformin side effects can include digestive issues such as gas, diarrhea, and vomiting. In rare cases, a buildup of metformin in the body has also been linked to lactic acidosis.

Statins

Statins are a type of medication that is frequently prescribed to reduce the amount of cholesterol in the bloodstream. Statins help to reduce the chances of having a heart attack, stroke, or dying from heart disease by lowering these cholesterol levels.

Statins work by lowering the level of C-reactive protein ("CRP") in the bloodstream. When the inflammatory response is activated, the liver reacts by releasing CRP into the bloodstream, where it can aid in the elimination of various pathogens. Statins can help to control and limit the body's inflammatory response by lowering CRP levels in the bloodstream.

Headache, rash, difficulty sleeping, constipation, flushing of the skin, diarrhea, muscle pain, bloating and/or gas, drowsiness, abdominal discomfort, dizziness, nausea, and vomiting are all common side effects of statins. Statins can also cause memory loss, high blood sugar, mental confusion, type 2 diabetes, neuropathy, myositis, rhabdomyolysis, and increased levels of creatine kinase ("CPK"), a muscle enzyme that, when elevated, can cause pain, weakness, and inflammation.

Anti-Histamines

Histamines are inflammatory hormones that the body produces. A "histamine" is a type of organic chemical compound that the body produces as part of its immune response to allergens, pathogens, or trauma. Histamines are responsible for ridding the body of the allergen that triggers the immune response. Histamines accomplish this by increasing the permeability of blood vessel walls, allowing antibodies, white blood cells, and fluids to flow out of the body's bloodstream and into the affected tissue. Inflammation results from the accumulation of all of these additional substances in the affected tissue. Histamines are thus essential for the immune system to function properly.

Anti-histamines, as the name implies, counteract the inflammatory effect of histamines, which, as previously stated, are responsible for initiating the inflammatory process. Antihistamines accomplish this by binding to inactive histamine receptors in your body, ensuring that those receptors remain inactive. Based on their effects on the central nervous system, antihistamines are classified as either first-generation (sedating) or second-generation (non-sedating). That is, antihistamines are classified based on whether or not they cause drowsiness.

Sedating antihistamines are most commonly used in low doses and for a short time in order to minimize the effects of inflammation that occurs as part of the body's allergic response and are not ordinarily used to treat systemic, chronic inflammation. However, non-sedating antihistamines tend to be used for a longer period, and in very rare instances, have been linked to mild and self-limiting liver injury. However, antihistamines are considered relatively safe and have been found to have only mild side effects associated with both short and long-term use.

Common medications include Zyrtec, Dimetapp, Benadryl, Chlor-Trimeton, Dramamine, Unisom, and Claritin.

Anti-histamines can also be found naturally. A few of these natural sources of anti-histamines are:

Vitamin C

Vitamin C is one of nature's most powerful antioxidants and anti-inflammatories. Vitamin C can be found in supplement form as well as in:

- Winter squash
- Broccoli
- Tomatoes and tomato juice
- Cauliflower
- Citrus fruits
- Cantaloupe
- Kiwi
- Strawberries
- Bell peppers

Probiotics

Probiotics are microorganisms that help fight off allergic inflammation by boosting the immune system and by assisting the gut in maintaining a healthy ratio of bacteria.

Quercetin

Quercetin is an antioxidant flavonoid that can be found in fruits such as apples, grapes, and berries; in vegetables such as broccoli, red onions, and peppers; in grains such as buckwheat and quinoa, and in fluids such as green teas, black teas, and red wines. However, Quercetin is more effective in supplement form, as the foods that contain it do contain a very small amount.

Bromelain

Bromelain is an enzyme that can be found in pineapples and in supplement form and is a natural remedy used to treat swelling and inflammation, particularly of the sinuses and that which occurs in the aftermath of an injury or surgery.

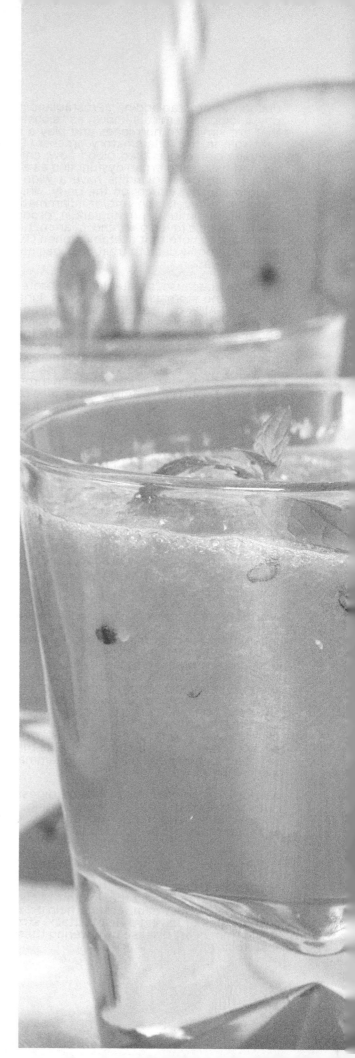

Chapter 5:

How to Build an Eating Plan Tailored to You

Meal preparation is an essential culinary tool for improving your overall health. Without a solid strategy in place, even the best intentions to eat well may prove futile. By following a menu plan, you can take charge of your health, reduce inflammation, and minimize your risk of illness. You'll feel more empowered, less stressed, and even excited about the tasty meals you'll prepare at home on a daily basis. Menu plans offer valuable organizational, culinary, and budgeting skills that are essential for a healthy diet. Once you understand how to eat in a way that works best for your body, you'll feel healthy, energized, and enthusiastic. And a well-planned menu can definitely help you achieve these goals!

Discovering the Best Way to Implement Anti-Inflammatory Action Plans for Your Needs

To ensure success, follow these helpful tips for making meal plans work for you. Schedule a specific time each week to go grocery shopping. Without making it a priority, meal planning won't happen. Choose a less hectic day to devote to purchasing and preparing supplies for your menu, which will help minimize stress. As soon as you can, prepare the ingredients for the coming week's recipes. Cut and wash vegetables in bulk, slice lemons, and cube meat. It's worth noting that most of the time spent on preparing meals is in the preparation phase, not the actual cooking. By doing this, you'll be well on your way to having delicious meals that are easy to prepare!

Get ready to cook by preparing some meals in advance, which can help alleviate the pressure of cooking during a busy week. For instance, you could make dinner for the first two days of the plan, cook a large batch of brown rice to use throughout the week, or prepare ingredients for your morning smoothie and freeze them in a jar, ready to blend the next day.

Seek support from family or friends, instead of doing it all by yourself. Ask your family, friends, or roommates to help with the cooking or prepa-

ration. It will help you complete the task more efficiently and make it more enjoyable. Encourage your children to get involved as well, as they can learn valuable skills that will benefit them later in life.

Make meal preparation and cooking enjoyable. Add some fun to the process by playing your favorite music, listening to a podcast, catching up on TV shows, or chatting with a friend on speakerphone. After completing the meal prep each week, reward yourself with a non-food treat like reading a good book or taking a walk on a beautiful day. Explore batch-cook recipes. As you follow your meal plan, you'll discover recipes you enjoy. Make double or triple batches of these dishes and freeze extra portions for later. Similarly, use dinner leftovers for tasty and nutritious lunches, or reheat a large batch of grains for an easy breakfast the next day.

Keep healthy snack options readily available. Hummus or nut-butter with celery and carrots, avocados, almonds, seeds, jicama sticks, and berries are all great options. Make extra batches of Mini Snack Muffins or Buckwheat Waffles, freeze them for quick reheating, and enjoy throughout the week in individual portions.

Don't give up if you find cooking daunting, tedious, or difficult, especially if you're not used to it. Like any skill, cooking improves with practice. As you continue with your meal planning and preparation, you will become more efficient and effective in the kitchen. You'll also start feeling more energetic and motivated to continue as you experience the benefits of a healthy diet. Each meal plan is designed to be anti-inflammatory, immune-boosting, good for digestion, and delicious. To help you choose the right plan for you, read on for an overview of each strategy.

The Plan to Get the Best from Your Anti-Inflammatory Diet

Regardless of the name, all anti-inflammatory diets advocate limiting added sugars and carbohydrates, eating less animal protein, and eating more fruits and vegetables. All anti-inflammatory diets are high in antioxidants, polyphenols, fiber, prebiotics, probiotics, and Omega-3 fatty acids.

While on this anti-inflammatory diet, you will be operating under the following principles:

- **Reduce or eliminate the consumption of processed foods and beverages.**

All processed foods and beverages contain added sugar and are the main sources of those sugars. As a result, by eliminating processed foods and beverages from your diet, you will also be eliminating the primary sources of those sugars.

- **Examine the ingredients on food labels.**

Reading the ingredient lists on food labels is critical to avoid all of the ways added sugars will try to sneak into your diet.

- **Make sure you're getting your anti-oxidants.**

Nuts, oily fish, raspberries, strawberries, blueberries, seeds, olive oil, avocadoes, sweet potatoes, beans, green tea, and dark green vegetables are high in antioxidants.

- Consume whole-grain carbohydrates.

Whole grain carbs are high in nutrients, such as fiber and antioxidants, which protect your body from inflammation. The zoo is a good place to start.

- **Consume more plants.**

"Plants," which include all fruits and vegetables, are high in vitamins, minerals, and antioxidants, which can all work together to protect your body from inflammation.

- **Supplements (optional)**

Anti-inflammatory properties have been demonstrated in a wide range of supplements. Taking supplements is optional because you will get all of your nutrients from the foods you eat on this anti-inflammatory diet. Before beginning any long-term supplement regimen, you should conduct thorough research and consult with a healthcare professional.

- **Consume Water**

Your body requires at least 64 oz of water per day to function properly. Also, because caffeine is a mild diuretic, your body requires eight oz of water for every eight oz of caffeine-containing beverage consumed.

- **Purple Grape Juice or Red Wine (optional)**

Red wine, when consumed in moderation, has been shown to reduce inflammation as well as the risks associated with heart disease. Drinking in "moderation" here means that a woman may consume no more than 5 oz (148 milliliters) of red wine per day and a man may consume no more than 10 oz (296 milliliters) of red wine per day.

If you do not or cannot drink wine, you can substitute it for purple grape juice.

- **Extra Virgin Olive Oil**

It is important to note that olive oil is only beneficial to your heart if consumed raw. Cooking changes the chemical composition of olive oil, transforming it into vegetable oil, which should be avoided. As a result, the majority of the recipes in this book use only a small amount of olive oil. If you use olive oil "in the raw," you can be more liberal with the amount you use.

- **Concentrate on Fish and Poultry**

Omega-3 fatty acids are abundant in poultry and fatty fish. Fatty fish should be eaten at least twice a week, with poultry and eggs providing the rest of the week's protein.

Fiber should be a key component of your anti-inflammatory diet plan. Fiber is beneficial to gut health. It also improves the body's insulin sensitivity.

- **Nutrient supplements must include fruits and vegetables.**

Those in search of the best nutrient supplements have every reason to give up. The majority of the nutrients required for a healthy body and mind are found in fruits and vegetables. They contain a lot of vitamins, minerals, and antioxidants. They are easy to digest and aid in the reduction of inflammation.

Every day, you should eat at least 4–5 servings of fruits and vegetables. Leafy greens, cruciferous vegetables, and fruits are all anti-inflammatory foods. Your anti-inflammatory diet will be inefficient and ineffective if you exclude them. They spice up your life and make you appear as healthy and energetic as they do.

- **Crucifers, when combined with onion, ginger, and garlic, can be extremely beneficial to your health.**

Add ginger, garlic, and onion to your recipes to increase their potency and flavor. They collaborate to fortify your immune system. Flavor can also be added to your dishes by using onion, ginger, and garlic. For flavor, you can also experiment with other spices.

- **More than 10% saturated fat consumption can be harmful.**

Saturated fats are bad for your health. They can increase the risk of heart disease and cause the release of free radicals. Consuming more than 20 grams of saturated fat per 2000 calories per day is not recommended.

Consumption of red meat must be reduced. It is difficult to digest and contains a lot of fat. To reduce the buildup of toxic compounds during cooking, marinate it with herbs, spices, vinegar, and fresh fruit juices before eating.

- **Omega-3 fatty acids are extremely important.**

Fruits, vegetables, seafood, and nuts are high in omega-3 fatty acids. You must eat enough of these foods on a daily basis. Omega-3 fatty acids are essential for lowering inflammation and the risk of chronic inflammation-related diseases. Cancer, arthritis, heart disease, and neurodegenerative disorders are just a few of the diseases that eating omega-3 fatty acids can help you avoid.

- **Increase your intake of cold-water fish.**

Omega-3 fatty acids are abundant in wild cold water fish such as salmon, mackerel, and trout. They also contain the majority of the other vitamins and minerals required. Consuming this type of fish on a daily or weekly basis will significantly improve your immunity. These fish provide all of the antioxidants needed for an anti-inflammatory diet. If you don't want to eat fish or can't find wild-caught cold-water fish, molecularly distilled fish oil supplements are an option. It would be a shame to miss out on either of the options.

- **Use healthy oils for the best results.**

Food may appear incomplete without oils and fat, but choosing the wrong oil can cost you a lot of money. Bad oil can harm your heart and promote free radical production. Your body requires fat, but it does not have to be bad fat.

There are many healthy oil alternatives, such as virgin and extra-virgin olive oil. You can also use expeller-pressed canola or sunflower oil. Polyphenols, which act as antioxidants, are abundant in these.

- **Physical activity is also necessary.**

A very significant fact that you must never forget is the importance of physical activity in your anti-inflammatory diet. Physical activity boosts your immune system and aids your body in its fight against inflammation. Your system can absorb the required nutrients fast and fight chronic illnesses better. Even small amounts of physical activity, such as a brisk walk, can aid in hormone regulation and maintaining a healthy balance. You will feel more revitalized and refreshed.

- **Reduce your sugar intake.**

This is critical to remember. When I say "sugar," I'm not just referring to table sugar. Refined carbohydrates are converted to sugar in the body. Refined carbohydrates include white bread, white rice, and French fries. The American Heart Association (2018) recommends that men consume approximately 9 tsp of sugar per day, while women consume approximately 6 tsp. I know chocolate and cookies are appealing, but we must resist and opt for fruit instead.

- **Reduce your dairy consumption.**

While fermented dairy products, such as yogurt, are generally safe to consume, fresh dairy products can cause inflammation on occasion.

Warning!

The initial days on an anti-inflammatory diet are not easy. In fact, the more necessary an anti-inflammatory diet is for you, the worse it will be. This is due to your body going through a withdrawal period in which it will be cleansing itself of waste and toxins. During the detox period, you are likely to experience a variety of cravings, mood swings, and possibly increased hunger.

Also, if you cannot drink alcohol in moderation, if you have a personal or family history of alcohol abuse or alcoholism, or if you currently have or have ever had any heart or liver disease, you should absolutely stay away from drinking any alcohol, including red wine. For the purposes of this anti-inflammatory diet, red wine can be substituted with purple grape juice.

The Protocol

The logic of this anti-inflammatory diet is simple: to reduce inflammation, eat less pro-inflammatory foods, and eat more anti-inflammatory foods. The idea is to affect a lifestyle change whereby your diet becomes based on foods that are nutrient-dense, contain plenty of anti-oxidants, and reduce inflammation.

Throughout your plan, you will be avoiding foods and beverages that are high in sugar, processed snacks, and meats, excessive consumption of alcohol as well as foods that contain a high amount of unhealthy fats and refined carbohydrates. This diet will provide a healthy balance of carbs, proteins, and fats at each meal.

The plan will give your body a chance to detoxify itself and thereby begin to recover from oxidative stress. It will also give your taste buds and appetite a chance to return to their natural state without being influenced by toxins found in most processed foods such as artificial sweeteners and hydrogenated fats. As a bonus, you may even lose a few lb

Chapter 6:

How to Do an Elimination Diet and Why AIP (autoimmune protocol) can help.

What is the AIP Protocol?

The Autoimmune Protocol, also known as the AIP diet, is a science-based diet that advocates for a complete diet and lifestyle change in order to manage and eventually send autoimmune diseases into remission. It is distinguished by a lifestyle change that necessitates the elimination of all inflammatory-causing foods in order to achieve deep gut healing of the leaky gut. To restore the balance required for healthy gut flora, inflammation-causing foods are replaced with nutrient-rich foods that address the body's hormonal imbalances and micronutrient deficiencies. Though the AIP diet is recommended for 90 days, it reduces inflammation within 15 days as the body begins to heal gradually.

It is critical to understand that all chronic and autoimmune diseases are caused by a "leaky gut" and its immune response, which causes symptoms such as hypothyroidism. As a result, eliminating the inflammatory foods eliminates the triggers that cause autoimmune symptoms and diseases. This eventually allows your gut, body, mind, and immune system to naturally calm and heal themselves.

Years of immune damage from eating foods low in essential nutrients and high in inflammation cause a serious imbalance in our gut flora. This causes a slew of negative health effects such as poor nutrient absorption, fungus and yeast overgrowth in the gut, and prolonged infections and recovery times. The AIP diet focuses on restoring the body's microbiome, which is made up of healthy bacteria that keep the body healthy. The diet promotes the consumption of high-quality probiotics, which are primarily derived from fermented foods and are high in healthy bacteria, bioavailable minerals, and vitamins that the body requires.

The AIP diet is a modified version of the Paleo diet that emphasizes nutrient density and the types of foods that should be avoided entirely. Some Paleo-approved foods are barred from the AIP diet because they contain compounds that may harm the gut environment and stimulate the immune system to attack itself. Nightshades such as peppers and tomatoes, alcohol, seeds, nuts, and eggs are among them. It should be noted that after some time, most of the eliminated foods that provide some nutritional benefit to the body but contain low amounts of harmful compounds can be systematically reintroduced.

The Autoimmune Protocol is a way of life that aims to manage autoimmune diseases by providing the body with nutrient-rich resources to regulate the immune system and promote tissue healing while eliminating inflammatory triggers. The AIP diet offers well-rounded and complete nutrition by avoiding processed foods, empty calories, and refined foods. In addition, the AIP lifestyle encourages stress management, adequate rest, and exercise to support immune modulation.

A leaky gut is required for the development of an autoimmune disease. Leaky gut is a condition in which the intestine's permeability increases due to the loosening of the intestinal wall junctions. Undigested food particles, toxins, and bacteria enter your bloodstream as a result.

What does this have to do with the food you eat? Some grain proteins, known as agglutinins, such as wheat germ agglutinin, and prolamins, such as gluten, cause intestinal permeability and promote the growth of harmful bacteria in the gut. Digestive enzyme inhibitors found in nuts, grains, dairy products, and legumes as well as phytic acid consumption, cause gut inflammation. Saponins found in nightshade vegetables, such as glycoalkaloids, are also harmful to gut health. Excessive alcohol and fructose consumption not only increases the likelihood of intestinal permeability but also harms the liver. These are some foods that the AIP diet avoids to improve gut health and thus manage autoimmune diseases.

Consume more vegetables to improve gut health and promote healing, especially non-starchy vegetables, which feed probiotic gut organisms. Foods high in vitamins K2, A, and D, as well as the amino acids glycine and glutamine, help to restore gut barrier function. Above all, maintaining an active lifestyle and lowering stress levels promote a healthy gut microbiome. The AIP diet recommends foods that promote the growth of beneficial gut microorganisms.

The AIP diet is intended to regulate hormones and, ultimately, the immune system as a whole. To regulate hormones, the AIP lifestyle encourages the consumption of specific foods, adequate rest, increased physical activity, and stress reduction.

By now, you must understand that the only way to regulate the immune system is by restoring a healthy level and diversity of gut microorganisms. This is done by offering the body substantial amounts of micronutrients and hormones that support a healthy and strong immune system.

How to Do an Elimination Diet

The elimination diet is a step-by-step process of removing specific foods from your diet in order to either determine which foods are causing you problems or to help alleviate symptoms from a current health condition. Once the foods have been identified and removed, it is clear to the individual what the trouble foods are and how they cause unwanted effects; as a result, diet followers can take the necessary steps to eliminate these foods from their diet entirely.

The main focus of the Elimination diet is getting key food groups out of your body. These include but are not limited to:

- Gluten
- Dairy
- Eggs
- Yeast
- Soy
- Wheat

Other foods you may want to remove from your diet could be citrus, nightshade vegetables, and nuts. The 'banned' foods are removed altogether throughout the diet and, towards the end of the dieting phase, are slowly added back so you can determine which specific item(s) is causing you all the trouble. As well as eliminating certain foods, you should also follow a controlled healthy diet high in plant fiber that can help reduce inflammation, a known precursor to many health conditions.

In addition to assisting individuals in eliminating food sensitivities, the elimination diet can also assist those looking to lose weight, with some people losing up to 20 lb in just one month!

Though some people recommend getting a food allergy test, these tests are not completely reliable and can sometimes be completely useless. The elimination diet is still one of the best ways to identify, remove, and completely eliminate problem foods from your life.

We are aware that not eating certain common foods, such as citrus fruits and certain vegetables, may pose a problem, particularly in a world with a growing restaurant culture; however, it will assist you in dramatically reducing your consumption of these foods if complete elimination proves to be a significant problem for your social life.

The duration of your elimination diet is usually determined by your age, overall health, and the severity of the symptoms caused by the food groups. If you're thinking about trying an elimination diet for your child, 7 to 10 days are usually sufficient. On the other hand, adults should stick to a diet for three to four weeks, though this can be extended if necessary.

Candidates for the elimination diet range from those with mild to severe allergies and sensitivities to those with more serious health conditions who would benefit from eliminating certain foods from their diet to alleviate the symptoms of their disease.

If you suffer from one or more of the following problems, then the elimination diet would be a wise choice to help mitigate unwanted symptoms:

- Asthma and other respiratory problems
- Autoimmune disorders
- Skin rashes
- Mild to severe arthritis
- Cardiovascular disease
- Mood Swings
- Attention Deficit Hyperactive Disorder (ADHD)
- Narcolepsy
- Headaches and more severe migraines
- Kidney abnormalities
- Insomnia and other sleep illnesses

You'd be surprised, but the list of conditions that could be affected by your diet is actually loner and continues to grow as more research is conducted into the area.

It is worth noting that the elimination diet is not restricted to those who just suffer from significant sensitives but can also be used by those who believe their gastrointestinal tract, digestive and excretion systems are not functioning as they should be.

The Elimination Diet: A Step-By-Step Process

The Elimination diet has three steps:

Step 1: Preparation and Planning

One of the most effective ways to achieve success with the elimination diet is to eliminate as many potential problem foods as possible. If you have a general idea of which food(s) is causing you problems, this may not be entirely necessary. It is also critical to keep a journal of all the foods you eat and all the foods you avoid so that you know exactly what your body is consuming.

Another purpose of the journal is to keep track of any lessened symptoms, changes in behavior or mood, and changes in energy levels. This makes it much easier to determine which foods are providing you with an extra boost. The elimination diet is an experiment in and of itself, and all proper experiments necessitate written results!

Everything boils down to preparation. To ensure you stay on the diet, you should plan in advance your meals and learn certain recipes to truly help you avoid the potential problem foods (some of which you may, unfortunately, enjoy eating). Know how to cook the foods you'll be eating; some may be unfamiliar to you, but give them a chance, and don't give up just because 'they don't taste as good.' Another excellent step before beginning the diet is to clear out the entire kitchen of processed and unhealthy foods and those you are removing from your diet. This will help remove any temptation to eat something you enjoy but is forbidden.

Step 2: Elimination

Though there are many variations of the elimination diet, with some foods being allowed and others not being so, below is an example of a potential diet routine. This one is quite restrictive, so if you're fairly certain that some of the banned foods do not cause you any problems, you may add them to your diet.

Fruits — You can eat many fresh fruits. You should, however, not eat citrus fruits (such as oranges, lemons, and grapefruit).

Vegetables — Virtually all vegetables are good to be eaten, however, when preparing them, try to steam, roast, sauté, or eat them raw. Vegetables you may want to avoid are tomatoes, sweet potatoes, and perhaps eggplant.

Starch — You should try to avoid as many starchy foods as possible, as these are known to cause many sensitivities and allergies. This could include rice. Starchy foods you should certainly keep out of reach are wheat, corn, barley, oats, rye, and products with gluten.

Nuts and Seeds — Nuts and seeds are very common causes of both minor and severe allergies and should be avoided altogether.

Legumes — Tofu, soy milk, virtually all beans, peas, and lentils should be eliminated from your diet.

Meat — Nearly all meat should be eliminated from your diet as it can have an impact on the functioning of the gastrointestinal tract. Many proponents of vegetarian diets argue clearly that humans aren't even designed to eat meat in the first place. If this proves too much of a problem, you could include turkey, lamb, and game.

Fish — Fish is generally not considered much of a problem for most people, so you are permitted to have a moderate amount.

Dairy — Virtually all dairy products should be eliminated from your diet. This includes milk, cottage cheese, cheese, eggs, cream, and ice cream. Alternatively, you can try including coconut milk or rice milk (without sweeteners); however, should you suspect a sensitivity to grains, rice milk should be banned as well.

Fats — You can include pressed olive oil, flaxseed oil, and coconut oil in your diet. However, eliminate all hydrogenated and processed fats such as margarine, butter, mayonnaise, and Caesar salad dressings.

Drinks and Beverages – While on the diet, or any restrictive diet for that matter, you should always consume large amounts of water, equating to nearly 2 liters a day.

Sweeteners — The only sweetener you should use is Stevia leaf. All others should be eliminated, whether they be white and brown sugar, high fructose corn syrup, corn, or maple syrup. This also applies to desserts, which you should not eat while on the diet, as they will inevitably be high in sugar, artificial ingredients, and calories.

Herbs and Spices — When on the elimination diet, you should try to use sea salt, freshly ground pepper, fresh herbs and other spices such as garlic, cumin, ginger, parsley, and turmeric. You should however completely avoid other condiments like mustard, ketchup, relish, BBQ sauce, soy sauce, and vinegar.

Step 3: Reintroduction of Foods into Your Diet

The elimination diet's goal is not to eliminate food groups from your diet for the rest of your life but rather to determine which foods are causing you problems. This is why you must gradually reintroduce certain foods one at a time in order to monitor your symptoms.

After 3 to 4 weeks of dieting, introduce one previously forbidden food and record your feelings, energy levels, and sleep patterns for the next 2 days. This process should be repeated until you have included all of the major food groups in your diet. If you experience any negative feelings along the way, you will be able to quickly determine which food is causing the issue.

The entire process of reintroducing foods can take up to 6 weeks, so it is important to be patient and remember the necessity of taking notes in your mini-experiment. Some of the key symptoms to look out for are:

- Tiredness
- Insomnia
- Brain fog
- Headaches and migraines
- Skin breakouts
- Bowel changes or stomach pains
- Exacerbation of respiratory problems

Reintroducing foods must be done in a systematic manner, gradually over a 3-day period for each food item. When common allergies are unknown, it may take three days for most people to experience a food reaction. Otherwise, it would be impossible to isolate all of the foods that do not belong in any given person's eating plan. You'll know which food item is to blame if you experience any side effects, such as fatigue, gastric upset, or headaches. When this occurs, discard the food item immediately.

When you reintroduce the food item into your diet, eat it 2 or 3 times per day for 3 days. You should also consume the food at various times of the day and for various meals. If eggs are being reintroduced, have one for breakfast, one in a salad for lunch, and one in a quiche for dinner. The foods that are being reintroduced should also be in their purest form, such as eating a fresh orange instead of drinking a glass of processed juice.

When returning dairy or gluten to the diet, only add one item from that category at a time, such as in the dairy category, by only adding eggs, not eggs and cheese. These two food groups contain the most allergens and cause the most non-allergy-related reactions in the body, such as achy joints and headaches.

Successful Elimination Diet users advise writing down any reactions to food items as they are reintroduced into your eating plan. These notes may be useful if, after the Final Phase of the diet, you notice no improvement in your mood or the inflammation in your body. Take these notes and observations to your healthcare provider so that additional analysis can be performed.

The best rule of thumb for adding foods back into the diet during the Final Phase of The Elimination Diet is — EAT WHOLE FOODS as much as possible!

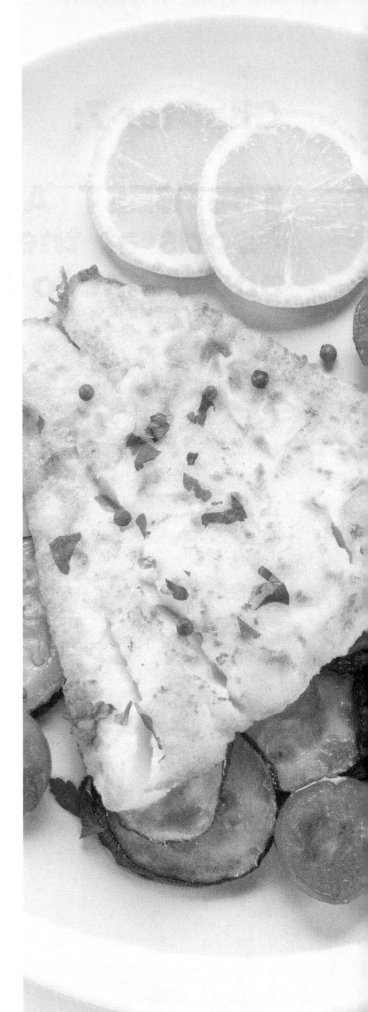

Chapter 7:

The BEST Anti-Inflammatory Foods at the Grocery Store... and What to Avoid!

Food List

Beverages

Eat in Abundance	Enjoy
Tea (Particularly Green Tea) • Water	Chai (with nondairy milk and no sugar) Coffee Kombucha Wine (limit 4 oz.)

Avoid or Minimize	
Beer	Liqueurs
Artificially or sugar sweetened drinks	Milk, dairy
Energy drinks	Soda, diet
Juice, sweetened	Soda, regular
Liquor, hard	Soft drinks, sweetened (with sugar or artificial sweetener)

Fruits

Eat in Abundance
Blueberries

Enjoy			
Chokecherry	Kumquat	Pluot	Santa Claus melon
Clementine	Lemon	Pomegranate	Satsuma
Coconut	Lime	Pomelo	Star fruit
Cranberry	Lychee	Prickly pear	Strawberry
Curran	Mandarin	Prunes	Tamarind
Date	Mango	Quince	Tangerine
Dragon fruit	Mangosteen	Raisin	Tayberry
Durian	Marionberry	Raspberry	Ugli fruit
Elderberry	Mulberry	Red currant	Watermelon
Fig	Nectarine	Salmonberry	Yuzu
Galia (melon)	Orange		
Goji berry	Olives		
Gooseberry	Papaya		
Grape	Passionfruit		
Grapefruit	Peach		
Guava	Pear		
Honeydew	Persian melon		
Horned melon	Persimmon		
Huckleberry	Pineapple		
Jackfruit	Plantain		
Kiwi	Plum		

Acai
Apple
Apricot
Asian pear
Avocado
Banana
Blackberry
Blackcurrant
Blood orange
Boysenberry
Breadfruit
Canary melon
Cantaloupe
Casaba melon
Charentais (melon)
Cherry

Avoid or Minimize
Processed juices with added sugar
Canned fruit in syrup

Grains and Starches

Enjoy					
Arrowroot	Buckwheat	Farro	Oats, rolled	Rye	Wheat, whole
Barley	Corn	Kamut	Quinoa	Teff	Wild rice
Bulgur	Cornstarch	Millet	Rice, brown	Wheat, cracked	

Avoid or Minimize	
Baked goods (bread, cookies, donuts, pies, etc.)	Pasta
Bread, white	Potato starch
Cereal	Rice, white
Flour, white	Wheat, refined
Oatmeal, instant, with sugar	

Grains and Starches

Enjoy					
Arrowroot	Buckwheat	Farro	Oats, rolled	Rye	Wheat, whole
Barley	Corn	Kamut	Quinoa	Teff	Wild rice
Bulgur	Cornstarch	Millet	Rice, brown	Wheat, cracked	

Avoid or Minimize	
Baked goods (bread, cookies, donuts, pies, etc.)	Pasta
Bread, white	Potato starch
Cereal	Rice, white
Flour, white	Wheat, refined
Oatmeal, instant, with sugar	

Dairy and Dairy Alternatives

Enjoy		
Almond milk, unsweetened	Hemp milk, unsweetened	Yogurt, coconut, plain, unsweetened
Coconut milk, lite, unsweetened	Kefir, water	Yogurt, almond, plain, unsweetened
Coconut milk, full-fat, unsweetened	Soymilk, unsweetened	Yogurt, dairy
		Yogurt, Greek

Avoid or Minimize			
Cheese, dairy (all types)	Goat's milk	Ice cream	Sour cream
Cow's milk (all types)	Half-and-half	Nondairy creamer	Whipped cream
Kefir, cow's milk	Heavy (whipping) cream		

Fats and Oils

Eat in Abundance
Extra-Virgin Olive Oil

Enjoy
Avocado oil
Coconut oil Macadamia oil

Avoid or Minimize	
Butter	Margarine
Canola oil	Palm oil
Corn oil	Peanut oil
Sesame oil	Safflower oil
Soybean oil	Shortening
Hydrogenated oils	Sunflower oil
Lite olive oil	Vegetable oil

Eat in Abundance
Salmon (and other fatty fish including tuna, mackerel, sardines, and trout)

Enjoy		
Anchovy	Eggs	Razor clams
Bass, wild-caught	Elk	Scallops
Beef, lean or very lean	Halibut	Shrimp
Bison, lean	Lamb, very lean cuts	Skate
Catfish, wild-caught	Mussels	Snapper
Chicken, free-range, skinless	Orange roughy	Sturgeon, wild-caught
Clams	Pork, boneless top loin chop	Tilapia, wild-caught
Cod	Pork, center loin chop	Turkey, free-range, skinless
Duck, free-range, skinless	Pork, rib chop	Venison
	Pork, sirloin roast	
	Pork, tenderloin (preferably pastured) Pork, top loin roast	

Avoid or Minimize			
Bacon	Chicken, fried	Ham	Pork, ground
Beef, feedlot	Cured meats	Heart (all types)	Salami
Beef, New York strip	Deli meats	Hot dogs	Sausage
Beef, prime rib	Farmed seafood	Kidney (all types)	Scallops, fried
Beef, rib eye	Fish, fried	Lamb, rack	Shrimp, fried
Bologna	Foie gras	Lamb, rib chops	Trout, fried
Brains (all types)	Gizzards	Liver (all types)	Whey protein
Catfish, fried			

Foods to Avoid Completely

The following foods are known to cause inflammation. Remove them from your regular diet and from your pantry shelves.

- Processed meats. They are high in saturated fats (sausage, hot dogs, burgers, steaks, etc.)
- Lard, margarine, and shortening are examples of unhealthy fats.
- Sugar-added products (except natural fruits): All canned sugar-added products such as soups, canned fruits, yogurt, bars, and so on.
- Commercial drinks, beverages, and fruit juices containing sugar.
- All packaged and processed foods. They have a lot of additives, artificial colors, and preservatives in them.
- White bread, white pasta, and noodles are examples of refined carbohydrates.
- Commercially processed foods, fried foods, candies, ice creams, and baked goods all contain trans fats (cookies, crackers, pastries, cakes, muffins, etc.) Beverages containing alcohol.

Chapter 8:

Tools and Tricks on How to Freeze and Store Food for Weekly Meals

What Is Freezing?

Freezing food is relatively simple because no special equipment is required, making it ideal for beginners. Before freezing, prepare your vegetables by blanching or cooking them. This process inhibits enzyme activity and ensures high quality.

This food preservation technique works well because microorganisms that could spoil food usually cannot thrive in temperatures -18°C (-0.4°F) or below. Additionally, the flavors of the frozen food items remain predominantly intact when thawed, while other food preservation techniques we've discussed often change or replace the original flavors. For example, drying intensifies the flavors of food items, while pickling infuses the brine or vinegar solution into the food.

The Fundamentals of Freezer Meal Prep

Traditional meal prep involves storing prepared food in the refrigerator, whereas freezer meal prep involves storing prepared food in the freezer. The advantage of freezer meal prep is that you can store food for longer periods of time than with traditional meal prep.

A large number of ingredients are being prepared for batch cooking.

Batch cooking entails preparing and cooking a large quantity of food in order to have leftovers. It can be as simple as making an extra serving of your family's favorite dish so you have leftovers for later in the week. Or you can make a large batch of soup, stew, or any freezer-friendly meal that you can then freeze, making dinner time easier on those busy days when cooking from scratch is difficult.

Benefits of Keeping Your Food Stash Frozen

1. Keeping your food frozen is a super-easy and effective method for preventing spoiling. When properly kept, frozen food can last for up to 12 months.
2. Frozen food items retain their flavors and nutritional value better and longer as compared to other food preservation techniques. In fact, many fresh products can be frozen immediately as these do not need to be cured or treated first.
3. All manner of food and drinks can be frozen. Aside from fresh produce, dried ingredients and pickled food can also be stored in the deep freeze after processing to extend their shelf lives further. Smoked and cured meats can last for years when frozen afterward. In many cases, cooked meals and leftovers can also be stored in the freezer to be easily reheated later.
4. Flash-frozen fresh produce undergoes minimal processing. This means that most frozen raw ingredients do not contain preservatives or other additives that may be detrimental to one's health. There is also no need to use salt or sugar to "improve" the taste or quality of frozen products. In fact, using these seasonings make frozen products deteriorate faster.
5. You can easily freeze seasonal fruits and store them for later use. This can save you a lot of money since you don't have to pay for pricey off-season fruits.
6. If you are not particularly fond of pickling or don't have the patience or equipment for drying or canning, freezing is one of the fastest yet most efficient ways of preserving your food. And, since most homeowners already have freezers in their kitchens, you do not need to buy additional equipment or tools.
7.

Equipment and Tools Needed for Freezing

- Freezer
- Freezer-safe storage containers or bags
- Freezer wrapping

There are loads of suitable wrappings and containers available to store your frozen food properly. Here are the most useful.

Clingfilm (Plastic Wrap)

You must use clingfilm that is suitable for the freezer. I recommend a multipurpose one, which can be used in the microwave and for other food wrapping too. Check that the film complies with the government recommendations for general food use.

Foil

Heavy-duty foil is best because it won't tear easily. Use it to cover foods as a lid over an open container, to wrap bread, meat, cakes, and other solid items completely, and to protect bone ends before wrapping in clingfilm or polythene bags. You can just twist and fold foil to secure it, but this must be done tightly, or the package will come undone. If necessary, seal with freezer tape. Foil is available in various widths and lengths in rolls or single sheets. The big advantage is that foods can be thawed and reheated in the foil if appropriate (but not in the microwave!).

Foil Containers

Rigid foil containers are ideal for storing everything from chunky soups to casseroles. You can also use them both for cooking and freezing prepared dishes, which can then be thawed and reheated in the same dish in a conventional oven. They usually come with foil-lined cardboard lids, which can be written on for easy labeling. Foil containers are designed to be disposable but sometimes can be reused; scrub very thoroughly to avoid contamination.

Foil bags

These are ideal for freezing liquids, such as soups or sauces, as they have a polythene lining and are very strong and leak-proof. (A cheaper alternative is to freeze the liquid in a polythene bag placed in a rigid container; you can then remove the rigid container once the contents are solid. Square or rectangular containers are best for this as they make frozen shapes that are easy to stack and store.)

Heavy-duty polythene bags

These are specially designed for freezing food and come in a variety of sizes, either loose or in rolls. I find it's useful to have a few small ones to hand for those little odds and ends you need to freeze, but on the whole, medium-sized bags, about 20 x 30 cm (8 x 12 in), are most useful for an average family. Experience will tell you what suits your requirements best.

Rigid containers

Made of polyethylene or other hard plastic, with airtight lids, these are ideal for storing liquids or semi-solid foods, such as casseroles and stewed fruit. They are also the best solution for freezing items that would get damaged easily in the freezer, such as a pavlova, cream cake, or delicate pastry (paste) dish.

Labels

As we have already seen, it is vital that you mark what the food is, the quantity, the date, and any special instructions for when it is thawed. Ordinary gummed labels won't do, as they won't stand the damp conditions; you must use self-adhesive ones with good sticking power. Freezer labels are widely available. Ensure you stick them on the bag or container when completely dry. If it's wet or greasy, they will come straight off!

Freezer thermometer

You don't have to have a thermometer, but it is useful to check the temperature inside your freezer from time to time. It should stay at −18°C/0°F.

What Are the Best Foods to Freeze?

- Stocks
- Soups
- Sauces
- Stews
- Bread and muffins
- Leafy greens and vegetables
- Sour cream
- Scrambled eggs
- Cooked pasta
- Cheese

Step-by-Step Freezing Strategy

1. **Wash, cut, and prepare the food you'll be freezing.**

You can freeze just about any food item or drink. However, there are a few that you should avoid freezing, including:

- Canned or tinned food items and drinks, or those in glass jars
- Cream pie fillings, custards, gravies, and sauces, unbaked cake batter, cake icin-

gs with egg whites, gelatin, and desserts that contain gelatin
- Fresh and boiled eggs
- Fried food items
- Mayonnaise and most condiments
- Raw potatoes and other tubers
- Cabbages, cucumbers, lettuces, onions, radishes

You should wash the majority of your food before freezing. This is particularly true for meat and seafood items. The cleaner the raw ingredients are, the less likely they will contain microorganisms that could spoil food.

However, high water content produce should not be washed. For example, fresh strawberries hold a lot of water. Once frozen, these fruits will expand greatly in size and collapse in shape and form as soon as they are thawed.

2. **Place food inside freezer safe container or bag and seal.**

I love the convenience of using freezer bags. They are easy to store before you use them since they don't take up much space and they're great for solid or liquid food.

You may also find it convenient to add a food label to your container with the contents as well as the data stored.

When adding food to the container, always make sure to leave some space for expansion. Due to the water content, frozen food and drinks always expand in size.

To avoid freezer burn (dehydration due to extreme temperature), make sure to use thicker freezer bags made especially for freezing and/or pre-wrap food in foil or saran wrap before placing it in the bag.

3. **Place the container with food into your freezer.**

The ideal freezing temperature is always 0°F or -17°C or less. If your freezer does not or cannot maintain this temperature, you can only store raw food items here for 2 weeks. After that, you need to cook them immediately.

4. **To ensure optimal flavor, always thaw frozen food items in the lower part of the refrigerator.**

True, this takes longer than thawing them out at room temperature. But the former allows uniform thawing.

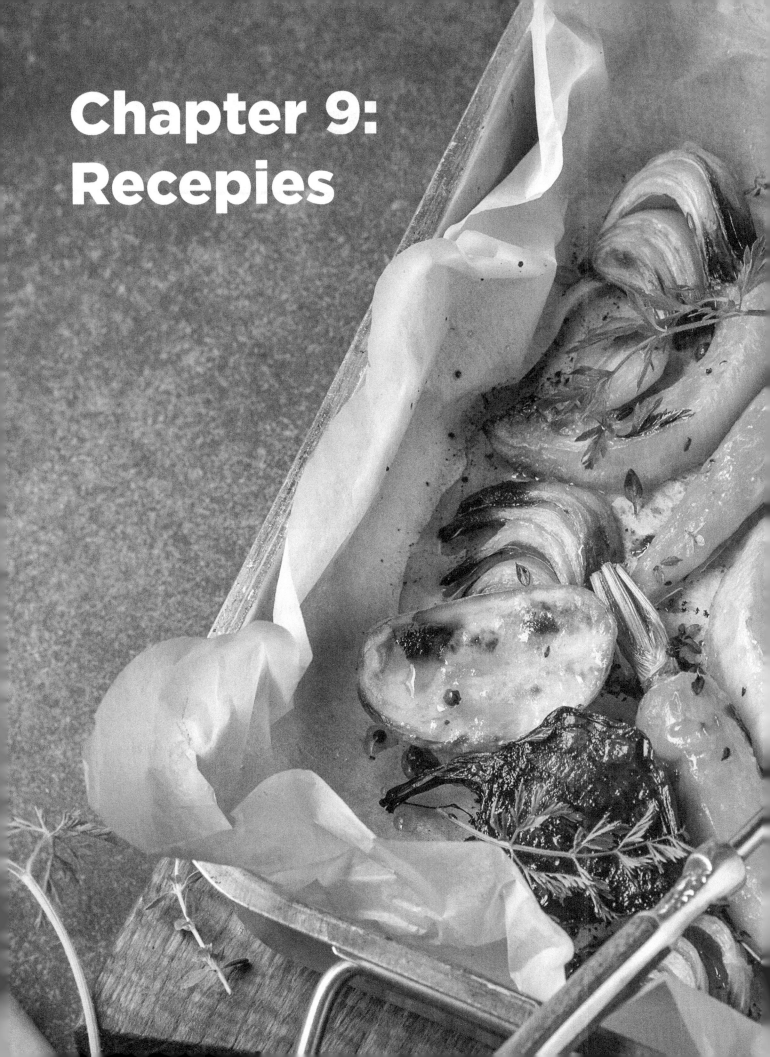

Chapter 9: Recepies

1. Berry Breakfast Shake

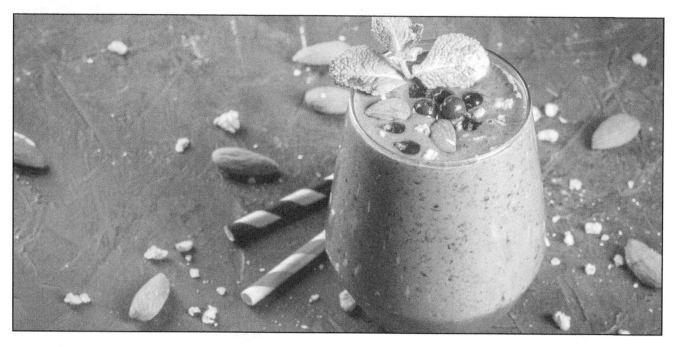

PREPARATION TIME: 15 minutes
COOKING TIME: 0 minutes
SERVINGS: 4
INGREDIENTS:
- 1 large green or red apple, peeled and sliced
- 1 Tbsp cacao powder
- 10 raisins, pitted
- 10 raspberries
- 2 cups blueberries, fresh and organic
- cup almonds, raw and chopped
- 2 Tbsp chia seeds

DIRECTIONS:
1. In a sealed container, add half the blueberries and apple.
2. Add the rest of the blueberries with raisins and raspberries separately. Then blend until smooth.
3. Add the blended mix to the apple and blueberries, and pour in the chia seeds.
4. Serve the mix and top with the crushed almonds and a dusting of cacao powder. It can be kept in a sealed container in the fridge for up to 2–3 days.

NUTRITION: Calories: 108; Carbs: 11.6 g; Protein: 3.2 g; Fat: 5.4 g.

2. Zucchini, Corn and Egg Casserole

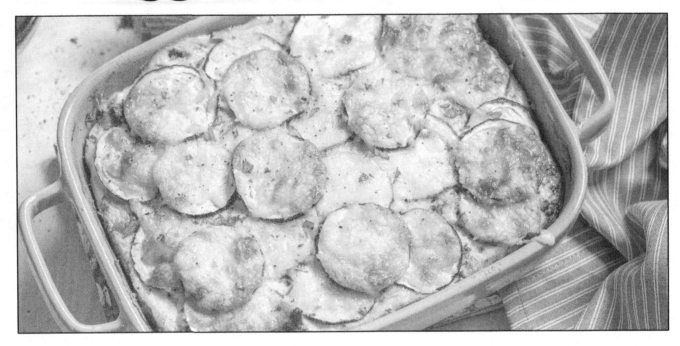

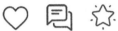

PREPARATION TIME: 10 minutes
COOKING TIME: 18 minutes
SERVINGS: 8
INGREDIENTS:

- 12 eggs
- ¼ cup water
- ¼ cup zucchini
- 4 cups spinach
- 1 can baby artichoke
- ¼ cup corn
- 1 Tbsp chives
- 1 Tbsp lemon juice
- ¾ tsp salt
- ½ tsp black pepper
- ¼ tsp garlic salt

DIRECTIONS:

1. Cover a round glass bowl with cooking spray.
2. Whisk the eggs and water in a medium bowl, then add the spinach, artichokes, corn, zucchini, chives and lemon juice.
3. Pour the mixture into the pan. In the inner pot, add 2 cups of water and the steam rack. Set the pan on the steam rack. Fix the lid. Set the timer to 18 minutes.
4. Quickly remove pressure until the float valve drops, then unlock the lid.
5. Allow it to cool for 5 minutes before slicing and serving.

NUTRITION: Calories: 133; Carbs: 6.5 g; Protein: 13.2 g; Fat: 6.1 g

3. Spinach Smoothie

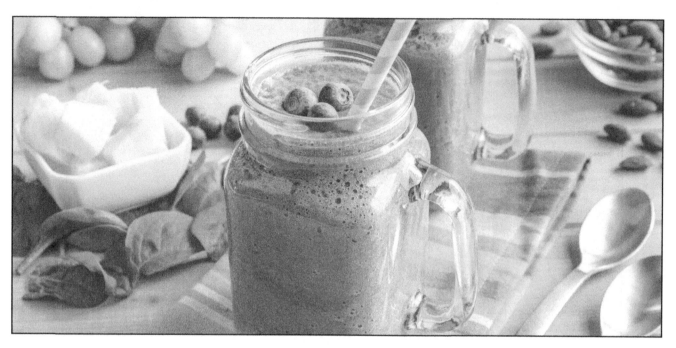

PREPARATION TIME: 15 minutes
COOKING TIME: 0 minutes
SERVINGS: 2
INGREDIENTS:
- 1 cup baby spinach
- 1 cup coconut milk
- 1 cup pineapple
- 1 cup ice

DIRECTIONS:
1. In a blender, place all the ingredients and blend until smooth.
2. Pour the smoothie into a glass and serve.

NUTRITION: Calories: 199; Carbs: 13.8 g; Protein: 2.2 g; Fat: 15.1 g.

4. Banana Oatmeal

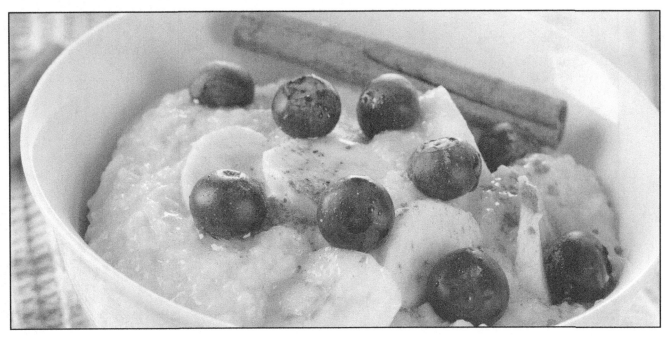

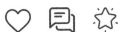 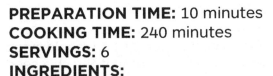

PREPARATION TIME: 10 minutes
COOKING TIME: 240 minutes
SERVINGS: 6
INGREDIENTS:
- 2 cups rolled oats
- ¼ cup almonds (toasted)
- ¼ cup walnuts
- ¼ cup pecans
- 2 Tbsp ground flax seeds
- 1 tsp ground ginger
- 1 tsp cinnamon
- ¼ tsp sea salt
- Butter
- 2 Tbsp coconut sugar
- ½ tsp baking powder
- 2 cups milk
- 2 bananas
- 1 cup fresh blueberries
- 1 Tbsp maple syrup
- 1 tsp vanilla extract
- ½ cup Yogurt plain

DIRECTIONS:
1. Mix nuts, flax seeds, baking powder, spices and coconut sugar.
2. Combine eggs, milk, maple syrup and vanilla essence.
3. Layer half of the bananas and blueberries in the slow cooker pot. Pour the milk mixture over the oats mixture.
4. Melting butter drizzle. Cook on low for 4 hours or high for 4 hours. Cook oats in liquid till golden brown. Warm it up and top it with plain Greek yogurt

NUTRITION: Calories: 310; Carbs: 40.6 g; Protein: 11.8 g; Fat: 11.2 g.

5. Chia Breakfast

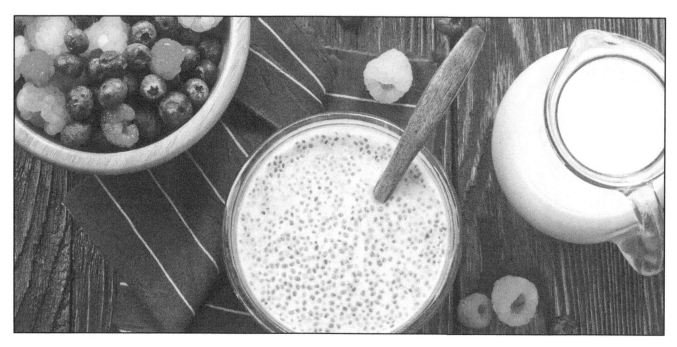

 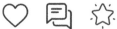

PREPARATION TIME: 15 minutes
COOKING TIME: 0 minutes
SERVINGS: 4
INGREDIENTS:

- • ¾ cup chia seeds
- • ½ cup hemp seeds
- • 2 ¼ cups coconut milk
- • ½ cup cranberries, dried
- • ¼ cup maple syrup

DIRECTIONS:

1. Stir together the chia seeds, hemp seeds, coconut milk, cranberries and maple syrup in a medium bowl. Ensure that the chia seeds are completely mixed with the milk.
2. Cover the bowl and refrigerate overnight.
3. Stir and serve in the morning.

NUTRITION: Calories: 272; Carbs: 7.5 g; Protein: 7.1 g; Fat: 23.8 g.

6. Greek Yogurt with Fresh Berries and Gra-

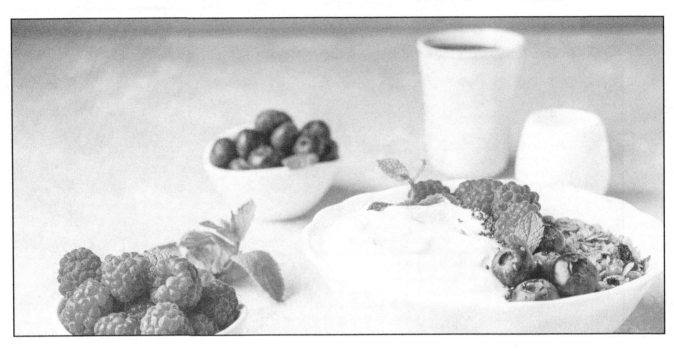

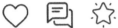

PREPARATION TIME: 10 minutes
COOKING TIME: 5 minutes
SERVINGS: 2
INGREDIENTS:
- 1 ½ tsp walnuts
- ⅓ cup Greek yogurt
- ⅓ cup mixed berries
- ⅓ cup granola
- 3 apricots

DIRECTIONS:
1. Pour yogurt into a bowl, mix in some apricots, granola and mixed berries, put in walnuts, and serve.

NUTRITION: Calories: 92; Carbs: 9.1 g; Protein: 7.9 g; Fat: 2.7 g.

7. Peaches Baked With Cream Cheese

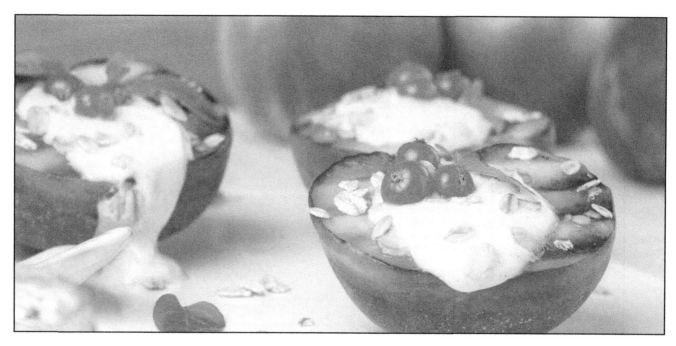

 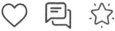   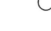

PREPARATION TIME: 10 minutes
COOKING TIME: 10 minutes
SERVINGS: 2
INGREDIENTS:

- 1 Tbsp extra-virgin olive oil
- 8 pecan
- mint sprigs for garnishing
- ⅓ cup cream cheese soft
- 4 peaches
- 2 Tbsp honey

DIRECTIONS:

1. Preheat the grill to med-high heat.
2. Brush the oil on the peach halves lightly. Place on the grill and grill for about 5–6 minutes.
3. Drizzle a little honey over your peaches and flip them over. In the center of each, put a scoop of cream cheese.
4. Cook for another 2–3 minutes until your filling is heated. Serve with halves of pecan and mint sprigs as a garnish.
5. Serve right away.

NUTRITION: Calories: 158; Carbs: 18.8 g; Protein: 3.8 g; Fat: 7.5

8. Baked Rice Porridge with Maple and Fruit

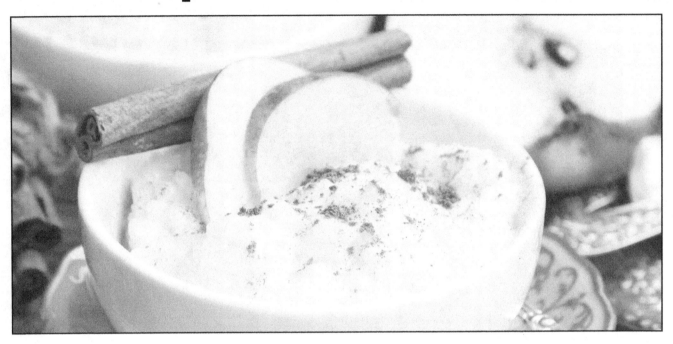

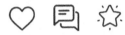

PREPARATION TIME: 10 minutes
COOKING TIME: 15 minutes
SERVINGS: 2 bowls
INGREDIENTS:

- ½ cup brown rice
- 2 Tbsp pure maple syrup
- ½ tsp pure vanilla extract
- Sliced fruits
- Pinch cinnamon
- Pinch salt

DIRECTIONS:

1. Preheat the oven to 400°F.
2. Boil 1 cup water and 1 cup brown rice in a medium saucepan. Mix in cinnamon and vanilla. Cover. Cool it down.
3. Cook the rice until done. Need to stir the rice? Use two oven-safe bowls. Put the rice evenly between dishes.
4. Put the cut fruit and maple syrup on the rice. Add salt. Bake for 15 min.
5. Serve

NUTRITION: Calories: 234; Carbs: 50.3 g; Protein: 5.4 g; Fat: 1.1 g.

9. Walnuts Granola for Breakfast

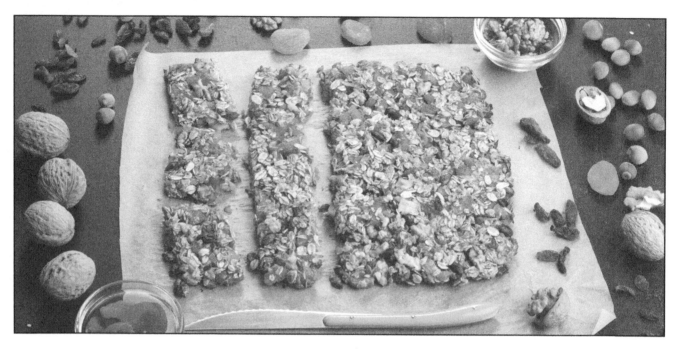

PREPARATION TIME: 10 minutes
COOKING TIME: 20 minutes
SERVINGS: 4
INGREDIENTS:

- 3 cups rolled oats
- ½ cup walnuts, chopped
- ¼ cup honey
- ¼ cup olive oil
- ¼ tsp ground cinnamon
- ¼ tsp ground ginger
- ¼ tsp ground turmeric
- ¼ tsp sea salt

DIRECTIONS:

1. Preheat the oven to 350°F.
2. In a large bowl, mix together oats, walnuts, honey, olive oil, cinnamon, ginger, turmeric and salt.
3. Spread the mixture onto a baking sheet lined with parchment paper.
4. Bake for 20 minutes, stirring every 5 minutes, until golden brown.
5. Let it cool before serving.

NUTRITION: Calories: 355; Carbs: 42.5 g; Protein: 12.4 g; Fat: 14.7 g.

10. Pumpkin Pancakes

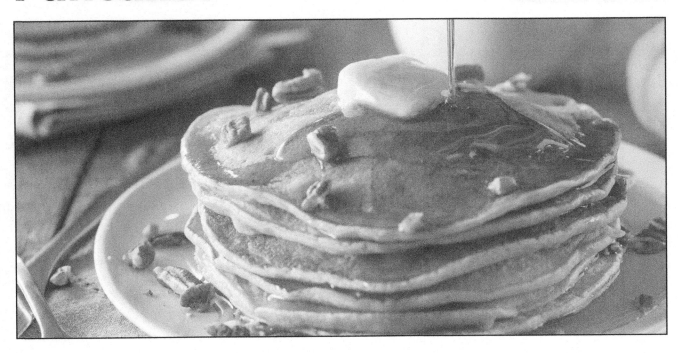

 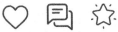

PREPARATION TIME: 5 minutes
COOKING TIME: 5 minutes
SERVINGS:1
INGREDIENTS:
- 1/5 lb egg whites
- 1 ½ Tbsp whole-wheat flour
- 1 oz pumpkin puree
- ½ tsp cinnamon
- 1 scoop protein collagen peptides
- 2 tsp stevia

DIRECTIONS:
1. Mix everything in a blender. Make it smooth.
2. Apply cooking spray to your pan. Heat over medium temperature.
3. Pour 1/3 of the batter into your pan. Spread evenly.
4. Cook for 2 minutes. The edges should be light brown.
5. Flip over and cook for another 2 minutes.
6. Sprinkle stevia on top before serving

NUTRITION: Calories: 258; Carbs: 24.3 g; Protein: 35.2 g; Fat: 2.2 g

11. Blueberry Breakfast Blend

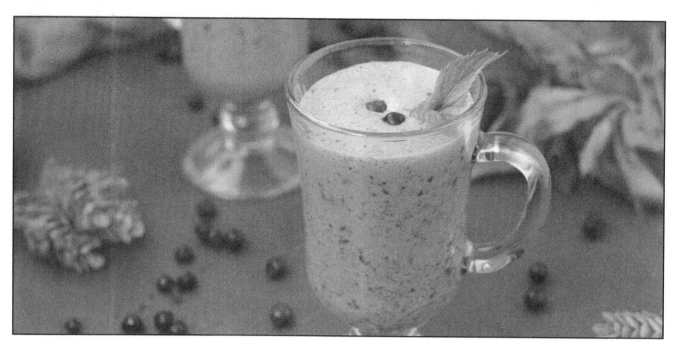

 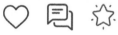

PREPARATION TIME: 8 minutes
COOKING TIME: 0 minutes
SERVINGS: 1
INGREDIENTS:
- ⅓ tsp turmeric
- ½ cup spinach
- ¾ cup fresh blueberries
- 1 cup fresh pineapple chunks
- 1 cup water
- 1 Tbsp chia seeds
- 1 Tbsp lemon juice

DIRECTIONS:
1. Combine all the ingredients in your blender. Blend into a smooth consistency

NUTRITION: Calories: 209; Carbs: 34.3 g; Protein: 6.1 g; Fat: 4.8 g.

12. Fruit and Millet Breakfast

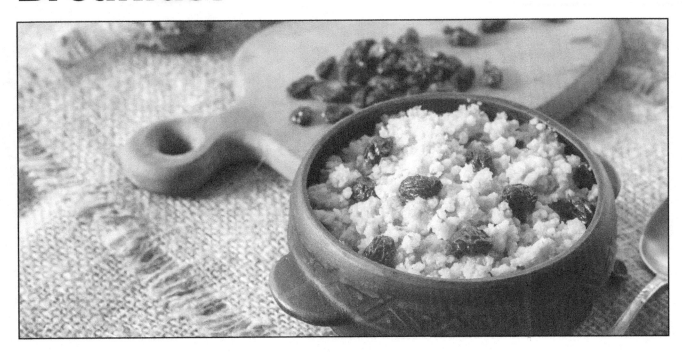

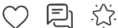

PREPARATION TIME: 30 minutes
COOKING TIME: 15 minutes
SERVINGS: 2
INGREDIENTS:
- ½ cup millet
- 1 cup water
- 2 Tbsp raisins
- 1 Tbsp currants
- ⅛ tsp cinnamon
- ⅛ tsp vanilla extract
- 1 cup coconut milk, unsweetened and divided
- 1 tsp honey
- ½ cup raspberries
- ½ cup blueberries
- 1 tsp hemp hearts
- 1 tsp chia seeds
- 1 tsp mint, chopped

DIRECTIONS:
1. Place the millet and water in a medium saucepan over medium heat.
2. Bring to a boil, and then add the raisins, currants, cinnamon and vanilla.
3. Cover with a lid, reduce heat to low, and let it cook for another 10 minutes until liquid is absorbed.
4. Turn the heat off and let it sit for 11 minutes.
5. Add coconut milk, honey, raspberries, blueberries, hemp hearts and chia seeds. Turn the heat to low and let it cook for 2 minutes.
6. Transfer to bowls and garnish with

NUTRITION: Calories: 329; Carbs: 42.4 g; Protein: 6.1 g; Fat: 14.8 g.

13. Veggie and Hummus Sandwich

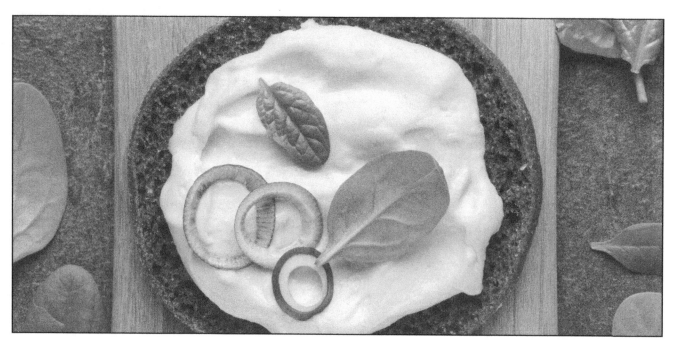

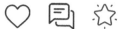

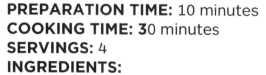

PREPARATION TIME: 10 minutes
COOKING TIME: 30 minutes
SERVINGS: 4
INGREDIENTS:

- 1 Tbsp Extra-virgin olive oil, plus additional for brushing
- 2 (15-oz, 425 g) cans garbanzo beans, drained and rinsed
- 2 Tbsp Chickpea flour
- ¼ cup tahini
- 2 garlic cloves, minced
- 4 scallions, minced
- 1 Tbsp Freshly squeezed lemon juice
- 2 Tbsp Lemon zest
- 1 tsp Salt

DIRECTIONS:
1. Preheat the oven to 375°F (190°C).
2. Use olive oil to brush a baking sheet.
3. Add the garbanzo beans, tahini, lemon juice, lemon zest, garlic and the remaining 1 Tbsp of olive oil into a food processor. Process until smooth. Then mix in the chickpea flour, scallions and salt. Pulse to combine.
4. Shape the mixture into four patties and put them on the prepared baking sheet. Put the sheet in the preheated oven and bake for 30 minutes.
5. Remove from the oven and serve.

NUTRITION: Calories: 321; Carbs: 41.3 g; Protein: 18.8 g; Fat: 9.0 g.

14. Black Bean Quinoa Bowl

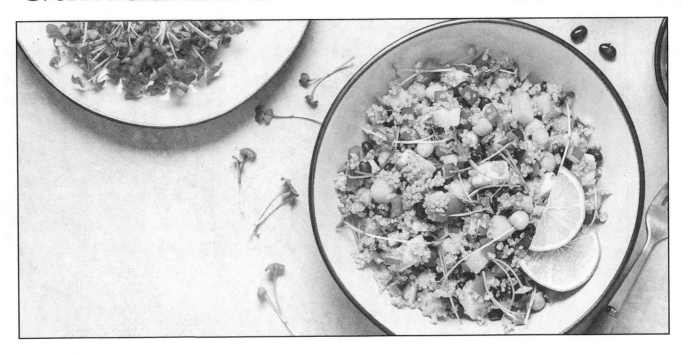

 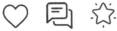   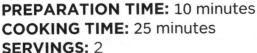

PREPARATION TIME: 10 minutes
COOKING TIME: 25 minutes
SERVINGS: 2
INGREDIENTS:

- 12 eggs
- ¼ cup water
- ¼ cup zucchini
- 4 cups spinach
- 1 can baby artichoke
- ¼ cup corn
- 1 Tbsp chives
- 1 Tbsp lemon juice
- ¾ tsp salt
- ½ tsp black pepper
- ¼ tsp garlic salt

DIRECTIONS:

1. Cover a round glass bowl with cooking spray.
2. Whisk the eggs and water in a medium bowl, then add the spinach, artichokes, corn, zucchini, chives and lemon juice.
3. Pour the mixture into the pan. In the inner pot, add 2 cups of water and the steam rack. Set the pan on the steam rack. Fix the lid. Set the timer to 18 minutes.
4. Quickly remove pressure until the float valve drops, then unlock the lid.
5. Allow it to cool for 5 minutes before slicing and serving.

NUTRITION: Calories: 133; Carbs: 6.5 g; Protein: 13.2 g; Fat: 6.1 g

15. Lentil Salad

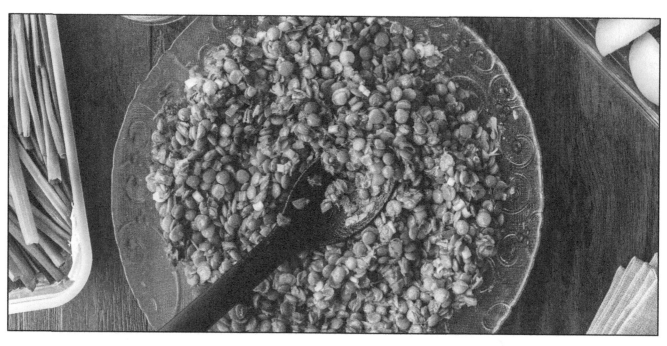

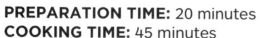

PREPARATION TIME: 20 minutes
COOKING TIME: 45 minutes
SERVINGS: 6
INGREDIENTS:

- 1 cup green lentils
- 4 cup water
- 1 cup quinoa
- 1 broccoli head
- 4 carrots, grated
- 1/3 cup extra-virgin olive oil
- 1 tsp salt

DIRECTIONS:

1. Rinse the lentils in a fine-mesh sieve. Add 2 cups water, transfer to a medium saucepan, and put over high heat. Bring the water to a boil.
2. Cook for 15 to 20 minutes or until the vegetables are soft. Any surplus liquid should be drained. Rinse the quinoa in a fine-mesh sieve.
3. Add the remaining 2 cups of water to another medium saucepan placed over high heat. Bring the water to a boil. Cook for 15 minutes or until the liquid is completely absorbed.
4. Allow cooling for 10 minutes after removing from the heat. Using a fork, fluff the mixture.
5. Combine the lentils, quinoa, broccoli and carrots in a large mixing basin. Add the olive oil and season with salt. If required, taste and adjust the seasoning.
6. Before serving, chill for at least 1 hour.

NUTRITION: Calories: 108; Carbs: 11.6 g; Protein: 3.2 g; Fat: 5.4 g.

16. Sandwiches With Green Salad, Avocado, Cucumber, and Cheese

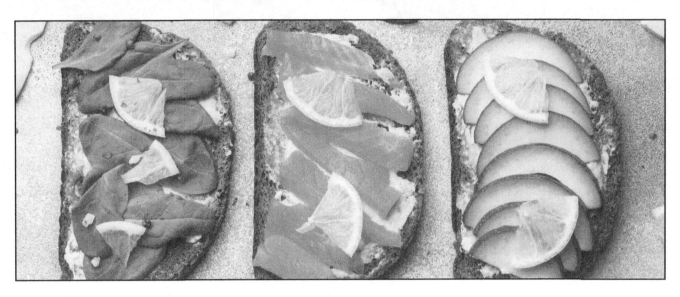

 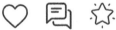

PREPARATION TIME: 10 minutes
COOKING TIME: 10 minutes
SERVINGS: 2
INGREDIENTS:

- 2 salmon fillets, skinless
- 2 cups seasonal greens
- ½ cup zucchini, sliced
- ½ avocado
- 1 cucumber
- Pepper, to taste
- 2 Tbsp cheese
- 1 Tbsp balsamic vinegar
- 1 Tbsp extra-virgin olive oil
- 2 sprigs thyme, torn from the stem
- 1 lemon, juiced

DIRECTIONS:

1. Preheat the broiler to medium-high heat.
2. For 10 minutes, broil the salmon on parchment paper with some oil, lemon, cheese, and pepper.
3. Slice the zucchini and sauté for 4–5 minutes with the oil in a pan on medium heat.
4. Build the salad by creating a bed of zucchini, avocado, and cucumber and topping it with flaked salmon.
5. Drizzle with balsamic vinegar and sprinkle with thyme.

NUTRITION: Calories: 387; Carbs: 7.6 g; Protein: 25.6 g; Fat: 28.2 g.

17. Veggie burgers with beans and vegetables

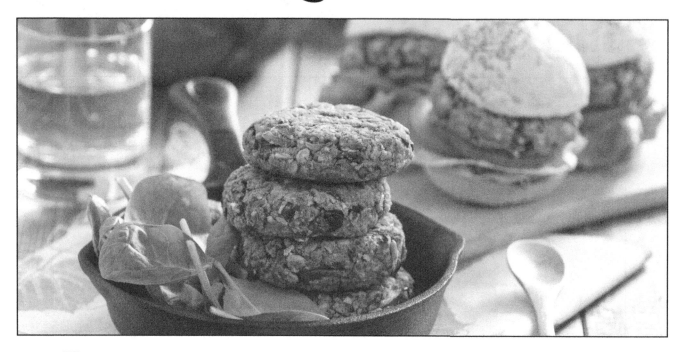

 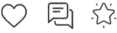

PREPARATION TIME: 10 minutes
COOKING TIME: 25 minutes
SERVINGS: 2
INGREDIENTS:
- 1 cup white beans canned
- 1 cup white rice cooked
- 1 tsp garlic powder
- ½ tsp chipotle pepper
- 2 tsp thyme
- ½ sweet onion
- ½ cup corn
- 1 big egg
- Juice 1 lemon
- ½ cup red pepper
- 1/3 cup flour
- Black pepper
- Salt to taste
- 2 tsp oil (olive)

DIRECTIONS:
1. Mash the beans using a potato masher in a mixing dish, making a few whole beans if desired.
2. Continuous stirring to integrate rice, thyme, chipotle, garlic powder, pepper, onion, bell pepper, corn, lemon, flour and egg. Season with salt and pepper.
3. Mold the material into four patties using your hands. Stir olive oil in a large pan over moderate heat.
4. Cook burgers for around 5 minutes on one side until browned, then turn and cook for another 5 minutes on the other side.

NUTRITION: Calories: 462; Carbs: 81.5 g; Protein: 19.4 g; Fat: 6.6 g.

18. Veggie Lunch Salad

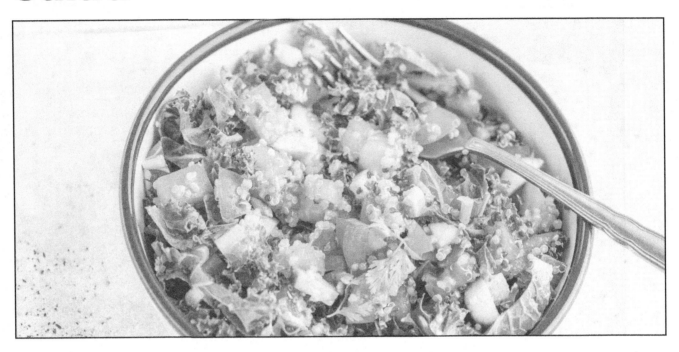

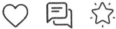

PREPARATION TIME: 10 minutes
COOKING TIME: 15 minutes
SERVINGS: 4
INGREDIENTS:

- 1 lb firm tofu, drained and cubed
- 2 Tbsp essential organic olive oil
- 12 oz yellow squash, cubed
- 2 orange sweet peppers, chopped
- ½ cup cooked quinoa
- ½ cup sorrel leaves, torn

DIRECTIONS:

1. Place a kitchen grill over medium-high heat, add tofu, grill for 5 minutes, and transfer it to your salad bowl.
2. Heat up a pan with all the oil over medium-high heat, add squash, peppers and quinoa, stir it, and cook for 10 minutes.
3. Transfer to the bowl with all the tofu, add sorrel leaves and Italian dressing, toss, and serve for lunch.
4. Enjoy!

NUTRITION: Calories: 202; Carbs: 21.3 g; Protein: 12.5 g; Fat: 7.6 g.

19. Healthy Golden Eggplant Fries

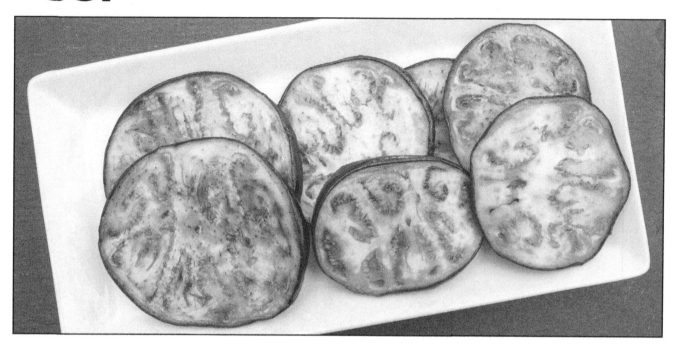

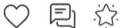 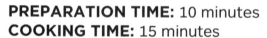

PREPARATION TIME: 10 minutes
COOKING TIME: 15 minutes
SERVINGS: 8
INGREDIENTS:

- 2 eggs
- Sunflower seeds and pepper as required
- 2 cups almond flour
- 2 Tbsp olive oil (for spray)
- 2 eggplants (peeled and cut thinly)

DIRECTIONS:

1. Preheat the oven to 400°F. Combine the almond flour, sunflower seeds and black pepper in a mixing dish. In a separate dish, whisk the eggs until foamy.
2. Put the eggplant slices in the flour mixture after dipping them in the eggs. After that, dip the eggplant in the egg, then in the flour.
3. Arrange the eggplants on a baking sheet that has been greased with coconut oil on top.
4. Preheat the oven to about 350°F and bake for 15 minutes.
5. Serve.

NUTRITION: Calories: 114; Carbs: 2.3 g; Protein: 4.6 g; Fat: 9.5 g.

20. Saucy Garlic Greens

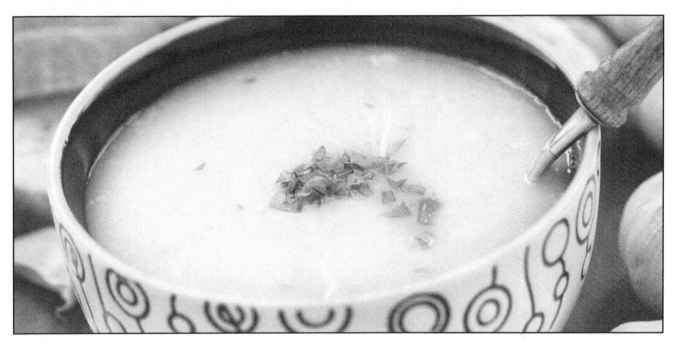

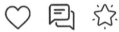

PREPARATION TIME: 5 minutes
COOKING TIME: 20 minutes
SERVINGS: 4
INGREDIENTS:
- ½ cup cashews
- ¼ cup water
- 1 Tbsp lemon juice
- 1 garlic clove peeled (the whole clove)
- 1 tsp coconut amino
- 1/8 tsp flavored vinegar
- 1 bunch leafy greens

DIRECTIONS:
1. Drain the soaking water of the cashews before blending them to create the sauce.
2. Freshwater, lemon juice, flavored vinegar, coconut amino and garlic are added to the mixture. Blend until a creamy cream forms, then transfer to a bowl.
3. Place a steamer basket on top of ½ cup of water in the pot. Fill the basket with the greens. Steam for 1 minute with the lid closed.
4. Release the pressure as soon as possible. Drain the excess water from the steamed greens in a sieve.
5. In a mixing basin, combine the greens. Toss in the lemon and garlic.
6. Serve.

NUTRITION: Calories: 86; Carbs: 5.3 g; Protein: 3.9 g; Fat: 5.5 g.

21. Delicious Vegetarian Lasagna

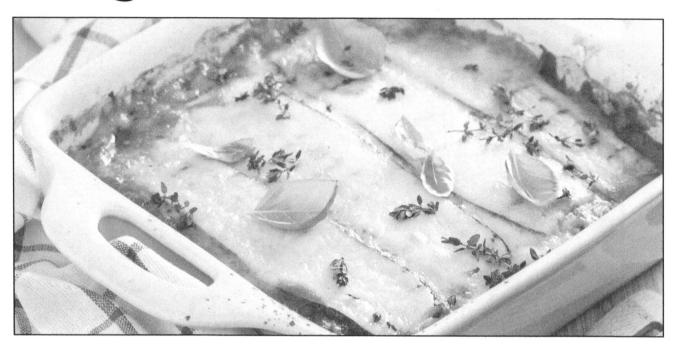

PREPARATION TIME: 10 minutes
COOKING TIME: 15 hour 15 minutes
SERVINGS: 4
INGREDIENTS:

- 1 tsp basil
- 1 cup sliced eggplant
- 1 Tbsp olive oil
- ½ sliced red pepper
- 2 lasagna sheets
- ¼ tsp black pepper
- 1 cup rice milk
- ½ diced red onion
- 1 minced garlic clove
- ½ sliced zucchini
- ½ pack soft tofu
- 1 tsp oregano

DIRECTIONS:

1. If using a gas oven, preheat the oven to 325°F. Vertically slice the zucchini, eggplant and pepper.
2. Blitz the rice milk and tofu together in a food processor until smooth. Remove from the mixer. Heat the oil, add the garlic and onions, and cook for 3–4 minutes, until tender.
3. Stir in the herbs (oregano) and pepper for 5–6 minutes or until the mixture is heated. Layer 1 lasagna sheet, 1/3 eggplant, 1/3 zucchini, 1/3 pepper and 1/3 white tofu sauce into a lasagna or similar oven dish. Continue with the following two layers, ending with the white sauce.
4. Bake for 40–50 minutes until the vegetables are tender and easily cut into portions.

NUTRITION: Calories: 222; Carbs: 25.0 g; Protein: 13.3 g; Fat: 7.7 g.

22. Chicken and Quinoa Salad with Spinach and Lettuce

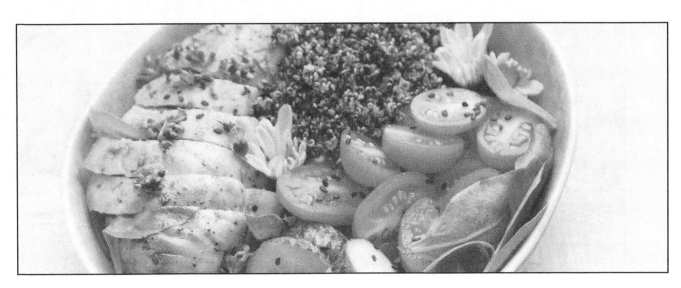

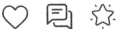 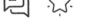 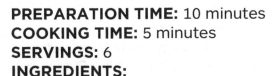

PREPARATION TIME: 10 minutes
COOKING TIME: 5 minutes
SERVINGS: 6
INGREDIENTS:

- 1 lb Chicken thighs (skinless, boneless)
- 1 can spinach
- 1 can lettuce
- 1 cup cooked quinoa
- 15 oz pinto beans (drained)
- 1 ½ cup cheddar cheese (grated

DIRECTIONS:

1. Heat the oil on medium heat with onions, then add the chicken and season with salt and pepper. Turn the cooker to low. With a fork and knife, shred the chicken.
2. Reheat the chicken with quinoa and pinto beans for 2 hours on low heat.
3. Cook and stir gently until the cheese melts. Add lettuce and spinach.
4. Serve.

NUTRITION: Calories: 314; Carbs: 33.2 g; Protein: 26.5 g; Fat: 8.3 g.

23. Grilled Salmon With White Bean Salad

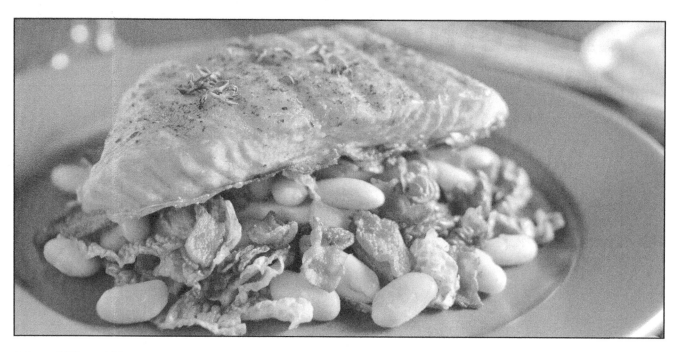

PREPARATION TIME: 10 minutes
COOKING TIME: 20 minutes
SERVINGS: 2
INGREDIENTS:
- ¾ cup white wine
- 2 Tbsp olive oil
- 1 Tbsp capers
- ½ tsp herb seasoning Mrs. Dash blend
- 2 8-oz salmon fillets
- 6 lemon slices
- 1 Tbsp fresh rosemary
- ½ cup White beans
- 6 Tbsp lemon juice
-

DIRECTIONS:
1. Brush with pepper, Mrs. Dash and minced rosemary, and spray the top and bottom of the salmon fillets using olive oil. Put every piece of salmon seasoned on a sheet of aluminum foil wide enough, just to roll over and seal.
2. Use 3 slices of lemon and 3 Tbsp of lemon juice, 2 Tbsp of wine, and ½ Tbsp of capers to top each portion.
3. Tightly seal the salmon in foil bags. Over medium heat, position a grill pan or heat it up a charcoal grill. Upon this hot grill, put foil packets and simmer for 10 minutes for a 1-inch slice of salmon. Mix white beans, lemon juice, rosemary and herb seasoning to make the salad.
4. Serve.

NUTRITION: Calories: 455; Carbs: 15.6 g; Protein: 36.4 g; Fat: 27.1 g.

24. Vegetable Spring Roll Wraps

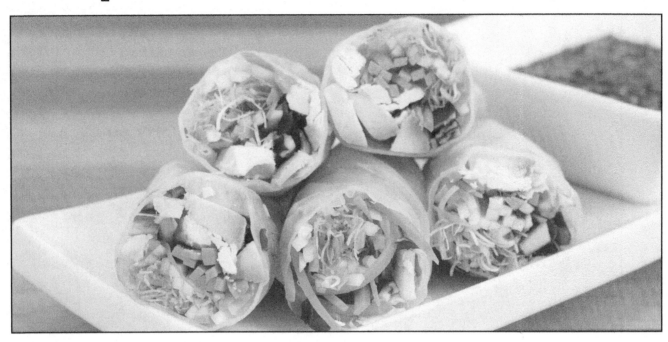

 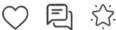

PREPARATION TIME: 20 minutes
COOKING TIME: 0 minutes
SERVINGS: 6
INGREDIENTS:

- 10 rice paper wrappers
- 2 cups baby spinach
- 1 cup grated carrot
- 1 cucumber (cut into thin, 4-inch-long strips)
- 1 avocado (cut into thin strips

DIRECTIONS:

1. Place the veggies in front of you on a chopping board on a level surface. Fill a large, shallow basin halfway with heated water — hot enough to fry the wrappers but not too hot to touch.
2. Every wrapper should be soaked in water before placing it on the cutting board, 2 cups of baby spinach, 2 Tbsp shredded carrot, a few cucumber slices and 1 or 2 avocado slices go into the wrapper's center.
3. Fold the sides over the center, then burrito-style roll the wrapper from the bottom (the side closest to you). Continue with the rest of the wrappers and veggies.
4. Serve right away.

NUTRITION: Calories: 69; Carbs: 7.5 g; Protein: 1.1 g; Fat: 3.5 g.

25. Curry Carrot Soup

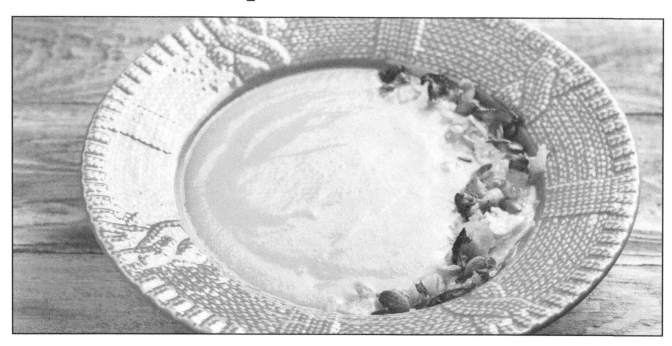

PREPARATION TIME: 10 minutes
COOKING TIME: 10 minutes
SERVINGS: 4
INGREDIENTS:
- 3 Tbsp essential olive oil
- 8 carrots, peeled and sliced
- 2 tsp curry powder
- A pinch salt
- 4 celery stalks, chopped
- 1 yellow onion, chopped
- 5 cups low-sodium chicken stock
- 1 Tbsp freshly squeezed lemon juice

DIRECTIONS:
1. Heat up a pot with all the oil, cook the curry powder over medium heat for just 2 minutes, add onion, celery and carrots, and stir and cook for 10 minutes.
2. Add the stock, stir, provide a simmer, and cook everything for 10 minutes more.
3. Blend the soup with an immersion blender, add fresh lemon juice, including a pinch of salt, stir, ladle into bowls and serve for lunch.
4. Enjoy!

NUTRITION: Calories: 154; Carbs: 10.8 g; Protein: 3.0 g; Fat: 10.9 g

26. Easy Broccoli Salad

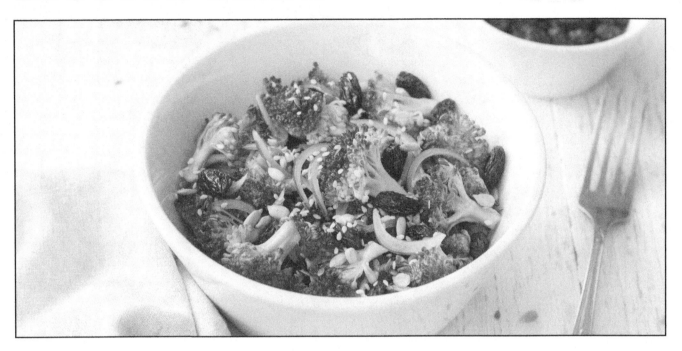

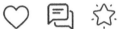   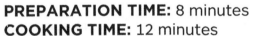

PREPARATION TIME: 8 minutes
COOKING TIME: 12 minutes
SERVINGS: 2
INGREDIENTS:
For the Salad:
- Salt
- 2 broccoli heads
- ½ cup Cheddar
- ½ red onion
- ½ cup almond
- 1 Tbsp fresh chives

For the dressing:
- ⅔ cup homemade mayonnaise
- 1 Tbsp apple cider
- 1 Tbsp mustard
- Salt

DIRECTIONS:
1. In a medium pot, heat 3 cups of salted water and then prepare a large bowl with ice water. Mix in the broccoli florets and cook until tender. Transfer it to the bowl with ice water after taking it out of the pan. Drain the broccoli when it cools down.
2. Blend all dressing ingredients and season well according to desired taste. Mix all the salad ingredients in a separate bowl and mix well until completely coated. Enjoy!

NUTRITION: Calories: 30.6; Carbs: 8.5 g; Protein: 14.0 g; Fat: 24.3 g.

27. Lemony Feta and Lentil Salad

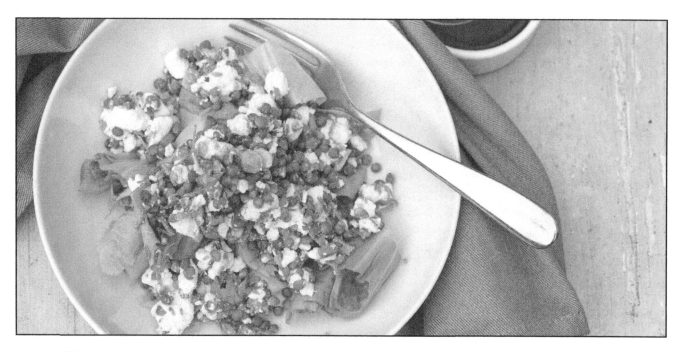

  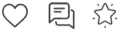

PREPARATION TIME: 15 minutes
COOKING TIME: 0 minutes
SERVINGS: 6
INGREDIENTS:

- ⅓ cup lemon juice
- ¼ tsp salt, or to taste
- ⅓ cup fresh dill, chopped
- 2 tsp Dijon mustard
- ⅓ cup olive oil, extra-virgin
- 2 cans (15-oz) lentils, rinsed, or 3 cups of brown/green lentils, cooked
- 1 cup feta cheese, crumbled
- 1 cup cucumber, diced
- 1 medium (red) bell pepper, diced
- ½ cup red onion, finely chopped
- Freshly ground pepper, to taste

DIRECTIONS:
1. In a big bowl, combine dill, mustard, lemon juice, pepper and salt. Whisk in oil gradually. Toss to combine feta, lentils, cucumber, bell pepper and onion.

NUTRITION: Calories: 286; Carbs: 33.4 g; Protein: 17.6 g; Fat: 9.2 g.

28. Tabbouleh

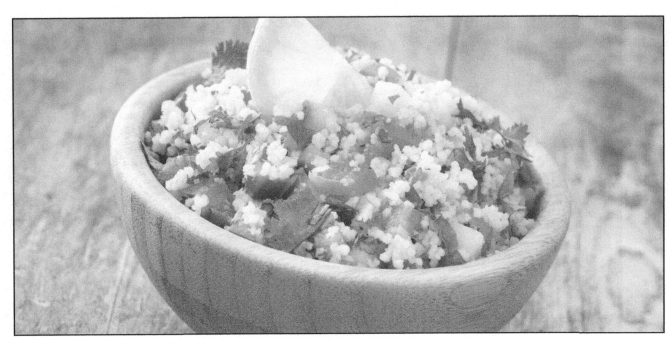

 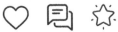

PREPARATION TIME: 25 minutes
COOKING TIME: 10 minutes
SERVINGS: 4
INGREDIENTS:
- 1 Parsley bunch
- 1 Mint bunch
- 1 Lemon Juice
- 3 Tbsp Olive oil
- ½ cup Bulgur wheat
- 2 medium Tomatoes
- ½ Red onion

DIRECTIONS:
1. Bulgur wheat should be soaked in 100 ml of boiling water for 5 minutes or until the water has completely been absorbed.
2. While doing so, finely cut the mint and parsley, and slice the red onion and tomatoes.
3. Combine the wheat with lemon juice, olive oil, herbs, onions, and tomatoes.

NUTRITION: Calories: 141; Carbs: 15.8 g; Protein: 2.6 g; Fat: 7.4 g.

29. Chicken Curry Served In Pan

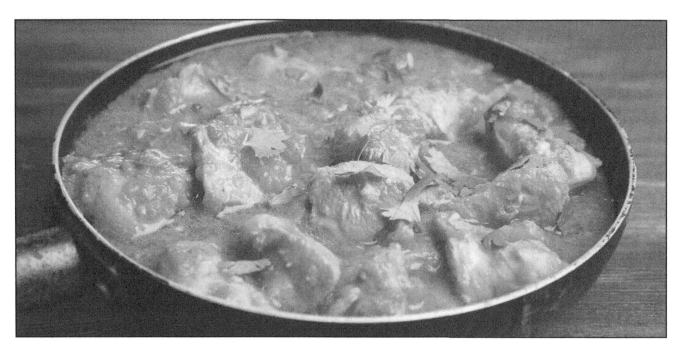

 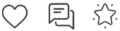

PREPARATION TIME: 10 minutes
COOKING TIME: 21 minutes
SERVINGS: 2
INGREDIENTS:
- 1 lb (454 g) chicken (skinless, diced)
- 1 Tbsp curry powder
- 1 clove garlic (crushed or garlic powder to taste)
- 1 medium onion (chopped)
- 1 tsp cornstarch
- 1 tsp canola oil
- Water as required
- ¼ tsp pepper
- 1 oz butter

DIRECTIONS:
1. Brown the onion and garlic in a skillet. In a tiny quantity of oil, add diced chicken and sauté slowly. Melt the butter in a separate pan and stir in the cornstarch. To make a paste, add a small amount of water. Whisk in the water (up to 1 cup), curry powder and pepper. Add the sauce to the chicken and cook until it thickens and reduces.
2. Reduce the heat to low, cover, and cook until the chicken is done. If necessary, add extra water to avoid scorching. With boiling rice or pasta, this recipe is wonderful

NUTRITION: Calories: 405; Carbs: 2.4 g; Protein: 42.2 g; Fat: 25.3 g.

30. Carrot Soup with Whole-Grain Croutons

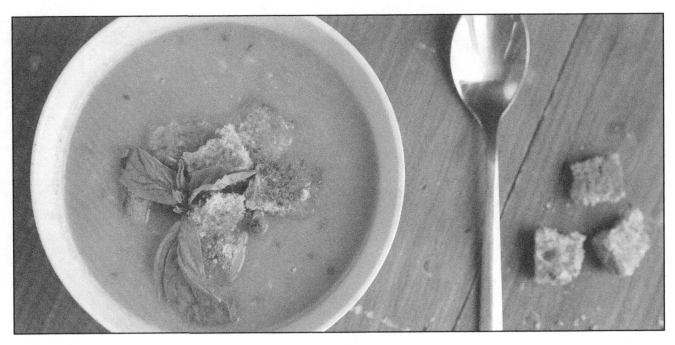

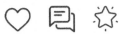

PREPARATION TIME: 10 minutes
COOKING TIME: 30 minutes
SERVINGS: 4
INGREDIENTS:
- 1 small-sized white chopped onion
- 1 Tbsp olive oil
- 2 Tbsp fresh ginger, chopped
- 1 chopped, cored, and peeled apple
- 1.5 cups almond milk, plain and unsweetened
- 4 large-sized carrots, chopped and peeled
- 8 oz canned no-salt chickpeas
- 4 cups no-salt vegetable broth
- 1.5 cups whole-grain croutons
- 3 tsp ground cinnamon

DIRECTIONS:
1. Heat up the olive oil in a big saucepan on medium heat. Combine the onion and ginger in a mixing bowl. Cook for 5 minutes, just until the onions are tender and translucent. Combine the apple, carrots, chickpeas, broth, whole-grain croutons and cinnamon in a large mixing bowl.
2. Cook the soup for 15 minutes or until the veggies are soft. Take the soup out from the heat and puree it in a mixer. Blend inside the almond milk until it is completely smooth. Alternatively, mix the veggies and also the almond milk in a saucepan with an immersion blender until smooth.

NUTRITION: Calories: 204; Carbs: 27.8 g; Protein: 10.3 g; Fat: 5.8 g.

31. Grilled Salmon Steak

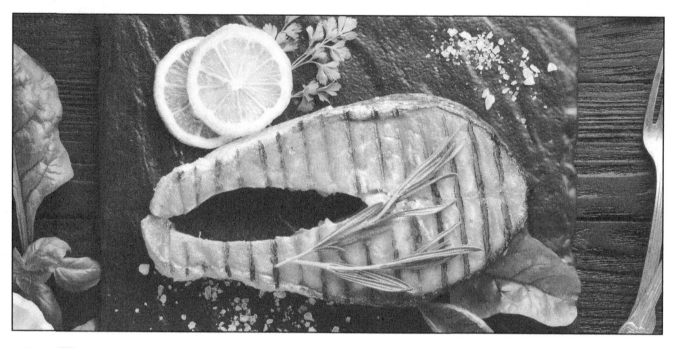

 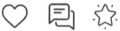

PREPARATION TIME: 10 minutes
COOKING TIME: 80 minutes
SERVINGS: 2
INGREDIENTS:

- 1 Tbsp fresh chives
- 10 black peppercorns whole
- 2 lemons
- 3 Tbsp fresh dill weed fresh
- 1 medium-sized onion
- 3 parsley sprigs
- 2 lb salmon steaks
- 2 bay leaves
- ½ tsp salt

DIRECTIONS:

1. Set aside one lemon in 6 wedges. ½ tsp of the zest of other lemon peel. 5 Tbsp of lemon extract. Cut the onion and chop the parsley and the dill grass.
2. Combine 2 Tbsp of dill herb, lemon zest chives and 1 Tbsp of lemon juice in a tiny mixing bowl for dressing. Cover and relax for a minimum of 1 hour.
3. Mix 1-½ cups of water in a 12-inch pan with bay leaves, 4 Tbsp of lemon juice, peppercorns, onion, parsley and salt remaining. Carry to a boil; incorporate the salmon steaks. Encompass; cook for 8–12 minutes or when measured with a fork, before the fish flakes easily. Serve the dressing-topped salmon steaks. Garnish with the leftover dill weed and lemon wedges.

NUTRITION: Calories: 398; Fat: 30 g; Net Carbs: 3 g; Protein: 28 g.

32. Farro Salad with Cucumbers

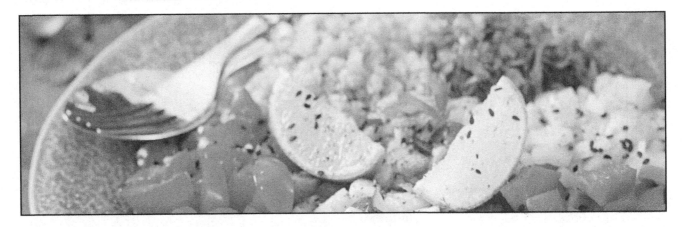

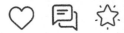

PREPARATION TIME: 10 minutes
COOKING TIME: 45 minutes
SERVINGS: 4
INGREDIENTS:
- ½ cup roasted chopped zucchini (see below)
- 2 cups Italian semi-pearled farro
- 1 cucumber
- 8 oz chopped fresh mozzarella cheese
- 1 (8-oz) jar roasted red peppers, chopped
- 2 Tbsp finely chopped fresh parsley
- 2 Tbsp finely chopped fresh basil
- 1/8 tsp dried marjoram
- Juice ½ lemon
- 2 Tbsp extra-virgin olive oil
- ¼ tsp sea salt
- ½ tsp cracked black pepper

Roasted Zucchini:
- 2 zucchini, cut lengthwise into ¼-inch slices
- 2 Tbsp extra virgin olive oil
- 4 Tbsp balsamic vinegar
- ¼ tsp cracked black pepper
- ½ tsp dried Italian herbs

DIRECTIONS:
1. Preheat your oven to 400°F for roasting the zucchini. Spray a cookie sheet using olive oil spray and place the zucchini slices on it.
2. After drizzling with olive oil and balsamic vinegar, top with pepper and dry herbs. Cook until zucchini begins to crumple and is soft and smooth, 8 to 10 minutes, on the center shelf of the oven.
3. In the meantime, boil a large saucepan of water, adding a splash of olive oil to keep the farro from clinging to the bottom. Cook in boiling water for around 30 minutes or until the farro is al dente.
4. 4. Using a strainer, strain the farro into a big mixing bowl. Toss the cooked farro with the cooked zucchini and other vegetables. Serve right after a thorough tossing.
5. 5. The mozzarella will melt if served warm but may also be served cool.

NUTRITION: Calories: 141; Carbs: 15.8 g; Protein: 2.6 g; Fat: 7.4 g.

33. Root Vegetable Loaf

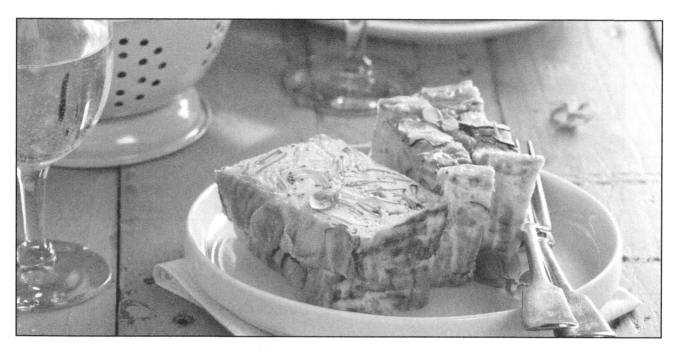

PREPARATION TIME: 20 minutes
COOKING TIME: 55 minutes
SERVINGS: 6 to 8
INGREDIENTS:
- 1 onion
- 2 Tbsp water
- 2 cups grated carrots
- 1 ½ cups sweet potatoes
- 1 ½ cups gluten-free rolled oats
- ¾ cup butternut squash purée
- 1 tsp salt

DIRECTIONS:
1. Preheat the oven to 350°F. Using parchment paper, line a loaf pan.
2. Sauté the onion in the water in a large saucepan over medium heat for approximately 5 minutes or until tender. Add the sweet potatoes and carrots. 2 minutes after cooking, take the saucepan off the heat.
3. Combine the oats, butternut squash purée and salt in a mixing bowl. Mix thoroughly. Press the mixture evenly into the loaf pan that has been prepared.
4. Bake for 50 to 55 minutes, uncovered, and in a preheated oven until the bread is firm and brown.
5. Allow 10 minutes to cool before slicing.

NUTRITION: Calories: 167; Carbs: 34.2 g; Protein: 4.5 g; Fat: 1.4 g

34. French Soup

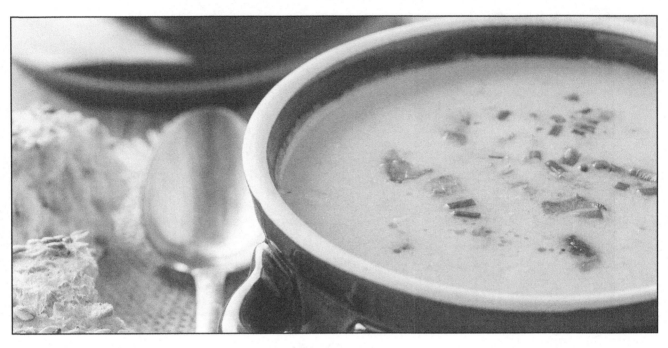

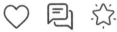

PREPARATION TIME: 10 minutes
COOKING TIME: 3 hours
SERVINGS: 4
INGREDIENTS:
- 2 Tbsp olive oil
- 5 yellow onions, cut into halves and then sliced
- Black pepper, to taste
- 5 cups vegetable stock
- ¼ tsp ground turmeric
- A pinch cayenne pepper
- 3 thyme springs, chopped
- 1 Tbsp tomato paste

DIRECTIONS:
1. Heat up a pot with the oil over medium-high heat, add onions and thyme, stir, and reduce heat to low.
2. Cover and cook for 30 minutes. Uncover the pot and cook the onions for 1 hour and 30 minutes more, stirring often.
3. Add tomato paste, cayenne, black pepper, turmeric and stock, stir, and simmer the soup for 1 hour more. Ladle the soup into bowls and serve.
4. Enjoy!

NUTRITION: Calories: 103; Carbs: 8.3 g; Protein: 4.1 g; Fat: 6.2 g.

35. Thai Cauliflower Rice Salad with Peanut Butter Sauce

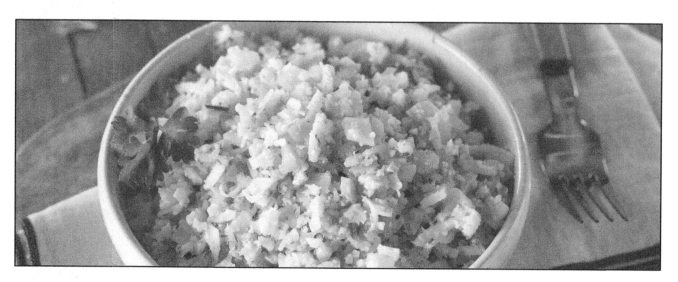

  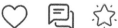

PREPARATION TIME: 20 minutes
COOKING TIME: 35 minutes
SERVINGS: 6
INGREDIENTS:
- 1 cauliflower (head)
- 1 cup coconut milk
- 1 onion (diced)
- 2 garlic cloves (minced)
- 1 fresh parsley (small bunch)
- 2 spring onions (chopped)
- ¼ cup almonds (toasted chopped)
- 1 peeled mango (small cubes)
- 1 bell pepper (small cubes)
- ½ cup red cabbage (chopped)
- 1 tsp coconut oil

For the sauce:
- 2 tbsp peanut butter
- 1 1-inch ginger piece peeled
- 2 tsp lime juice
- 1 tsp raw honey
- ¼ cup water
- ½ tsp sea salt

DIRECTIONS:
1. The cauliflower greens should be removed, divided into florets, rinsed, and well drained.
2. In a food processor, blend or pulse the florets until they resemble rice in size.
3. The garlic and onions are added to the hot coconut oil and cooked for 1 minute.
4. Add the cauliflower and coconut milk, stir, and simmer for 5 minutes on low heat or until tender but not mushy.
5. Please remove it from the fire and let it cool.
6. Combine mango, cauliflower, bell pepper, spring onion, parsley and red cabbage in a mixing dish.
7. In a blender, combine the sauce ingredients and pulse until creamy and smooth.
8. Pour over the cauliflower salad, then gently fold it in.
9. Serve after adding fresh parsley and almonds as a garnish.

NUTRITION: Calories: 167; Carbs: 34.2 g; Protein: 4.5 g; Fat: 1.4 g

36. Hearty Black Bean Soup

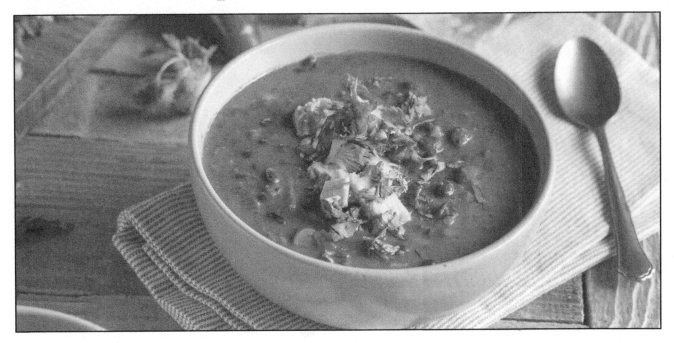

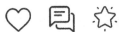

PREPARATION TIME: 10 minutes
COOKING TIME: 20 minutes
SERVINGS: 4
INGREDIENTS:

- 2 tsp organic olive oil
- 1 yellow onion, chopped
- 1 tsp cinnamon powder
- 38 oz canned black beans, no-salt-added, drained and rinsed
- 32 oz low-sodium chicken stock
- 1 sweet potato, chopped

DIRECTIONS:

1. Heat up a pot using the oil over medium heat, add onion and cinnamon, stir, and cook for 6 minutes.
2. Add black beans, stock and sweet potato, stir, cooking for 14 minutes, puree utilizing an immersion blender, divide into bowls, and serve for lunch.
3. Enjoy!

NUTRITION: Calories: 409; Carbs: 66.3 g; Protein: 27.5 g; Fat: 3.8 g.

37. Parmesan-Crusted Scallops and Greens

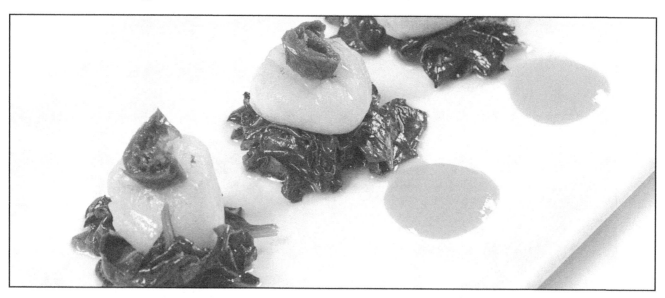

PREPARATION TIME: 10 minutes
COOKING TIME: 15 minutes
SERVINGS: 4
INGREDIENTS:

- 1 lb raw jumbo sea scallops
- ¼ cup cornstarch
- 1 large egg
- ½ cup grated Parmesan cheese
- ½ tsp dried or chopped fresh parsley
- 2 Tbsp extra-virgin olive oil
- 2 cups baby spinach leaves
- 1 tsp Salt - Freshly ground black pepper

DIRECTIONS:

1. Blot the scallops dry with a paper towel. Leave a bit of moisture on the scallops so the cornstarch will stick but not too much or the batter will not adhere as well.
2. Place the cornstarch in one small bowl. Beat an egg in another small bowl. Combine the Parmesan cheese and parsley on a medium plate.
3. In a medium skillet, warm the oil over medium heat.
4. One at a time, lightly coat each scallop with cornstarch on both flat sides, dip both sides in the egg, and then coat in the cheese and parsley mixture and set aside. Repeat for all the scallops, then place the scallops in the hot skillet. Cook on each side until golden brown. Remove from the heat and set aside.
5. Lower the heat to medium and place the spinach in the skillet. Cook for 3 to 5 minutes or until spinach is wilted. Sprinkle with salt and pepper to taste.
6. Serve the scallops over the spinach.

NUTRITION: Calories: 167; Carbs: 34.2 g; Protein: 4.5 g; Fat: 1.4 g

38. Alkaline Chili

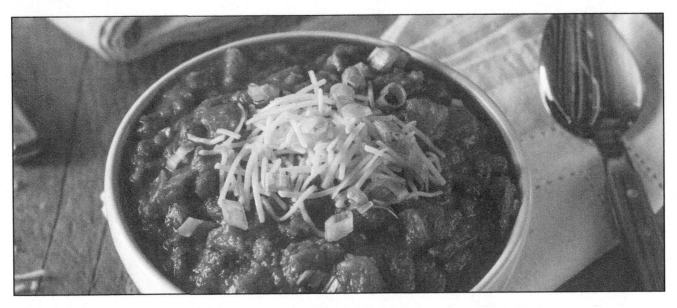

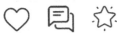

PREPARATION TIME: 20 minutes
COOKING TIME: 20 minutes
SERVINGS: 2
INGREDIENTS:

- 1 Tbsp olive oil
- 1 onion (chopped)
- 1 crushed garlic clove
- 1 can chopped tomatoes
- 2 Tbsp tomato puree
- 1 red chili, thinly sliced,
- ½ tsp ground cumin
- ½ tsp ground coriander
- q.b bragg Liquid Aminos
- ½ veg stock (yeast-free) cube
- Himalayan Salt and black pepper (freshly ground)
- ½ lb can red kidney drained beans
- 1 head chopped broccoli
- 1 handful spinach
- q.b. Lime wedges to serve

DIRECTIONS:

1. 1. Cook the garlic and onion until they are soft in 50 ml of simmering water or stock in a large, heavy pot.
2. 2. Cumin, Bragg Liquid Aminos sauce, powdered coriander and the crushed stock cube should all be added to the mixture along with the tomato puree, diced tomatoes and cumin. To thoroughly blend, stir.
3. 3. Salt and pepper to taste should be used liberally. Cook the mixture for about 20 minutes, occasionally stirring with a wooden spoon, at a moderate simmer, until it is rich and thickened.
4. 4. Include kidney beans and fresh coriander. Before turning off the heat and adding flavorings to taste, simmer under cover for an additional 8 minutes.
5. 5. After cooling, add fresh broccoli, spinach, raw and diced, and a little olive oil.
6. 6. This recipe pairs wonderfully with lime wedges, rice, guacamole and a large green salad.

NUTRITION: Calories: 232; Carbs: 32.5 g; Protein: 12.1 g; Fat: 5.8 g.

39. The Healthy Fish Tacos

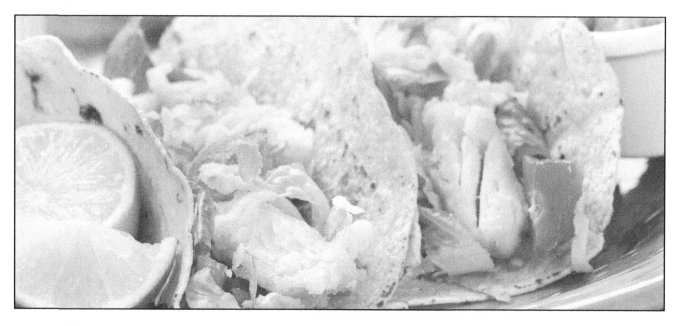

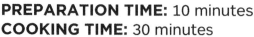

PREPARATION TIME: 10 minutes
COOKING TIME: 30 minutes
SERVINGS: 6
INGREDIENTS:

- ¼ cup olive oil
- 1 tsp ground cardamom
- 1 tsp paprika
- 1 tsp salt
- 1 tsp pepper
- 6 fillets mahi-mahi (6 oz each)
- 12 (6") corn tortillas
- 2 cups red cabbage chopped
- 1 cup fresh cilantro chopped
- Salsa verde
- 2 wedged medium limes
- Tapatio sauce

DIRECTIONS:

1. Combine the first five ingredients in a 13 by 9-inch baking dish. Add the fish fillets and marinate them well.
2. Refrigerate for approximately half an hour, covered. Remove the fish from the marinade and discard it. Place the fillets on the oiled grilling rack and cover them.
3. Grill them over medium-high heat for approximately 5 minutes on each side or until they can easily be flaked with a fork. Remove the fillets from the grill and set them aside.
4. For approximately half a minute, heat the tortillas. Arrange the red cabbage, salsa verde and cilantro on top of the fish, which has been divided into equal halves.
5. Squeeze a little lime juice and a dash of spicy sauce over the top. Fold the edges of the bag over the fish fillets.
6. Serve with more pepper sauce plus lemon wedges on the side.

NUTRITION: Calories: 339; Carbs: 26.1 g; Protein: 34.8 g; Fat: 10.4 g.

40. Cod Fillet With Herbs

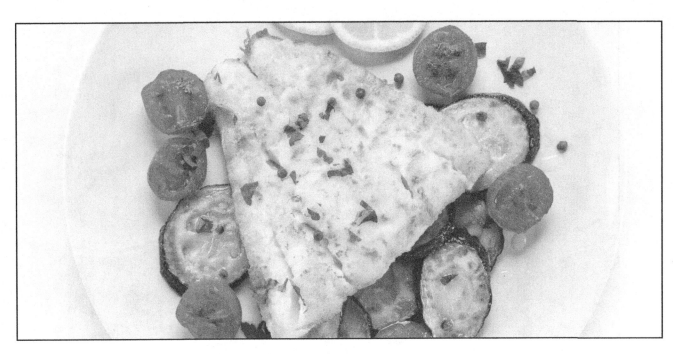

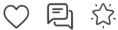

PREPARATION TIME: 10 minutes
COOKING TIME: 25 minutes
SERVINGS: 2
INGREDIENTS:

- 2 cups mustard greens
- 1 lb skinless cod fillet
- ½ zucchini, sliced
- 2 Tbsp extra-virgin olive oil
- 2 Tbsp Mixed herbs
- 2 thyme sprigs, torn
- 1 lemon, juiced

DIRECTIONS:

1. Brush the cod fillet with olive oil and fry it in a pan over medium heat until browned. Remove and flake it.
2. Sauté the zucchini and mustard greens in the same pan for 4–5 minutes. Transfer to a plate and top with cod.
3. Drizzle with lemon and sprinkle with thyme and Mixed herbs.
4. Serve

NUTRITION: Calories: 360; Carbs: 6.5 g; Protein: 37.6 g; Fat: 20.3 g

41. Roasted Cauliflower With Cheese

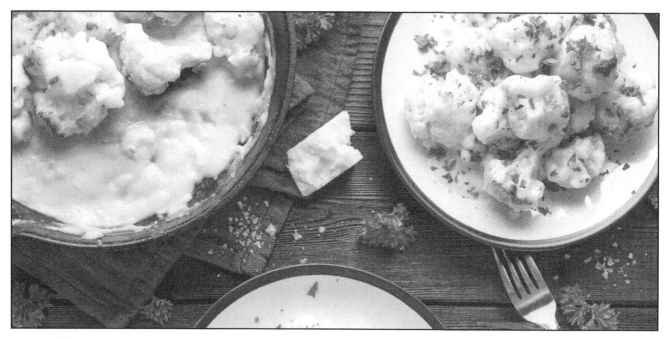

 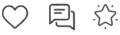

PREPARATION TIME: 10 minutes
COOKING TIME: 40 minutes
SERVINGS: 2
INGREDIENTS:
- 3 cups cauliflower florets
- 1/3 cup Tahini
- 1/5 cup extra-virgin olive oil
- 2 Tbsp lemon juice
- 2 Tbsp cheddar cheese
- 1 garlic clove
- 1/3 tsp paprika
- ¾ tsp salt
- Water
- ¼ tsp black pepper

DIRECTIONS:
1. Preheat your oven to a temperature of 390°F. Line parchment paper in a baking pan, arrange the cauliflower and add cheese.
2. Drizzle with 2 Tbsp of oil and season with black pepper and salt. Roast for around 30 minutes.
3. Process in a blender with the rest of the ingredients and serve at room temperature.

NUTRITION: Calories: 339; Carbs: 26.1 g; Protein: 34.8 g; Fat: 10.4 g.

42. Mexican Quinoa and Lemon Salad

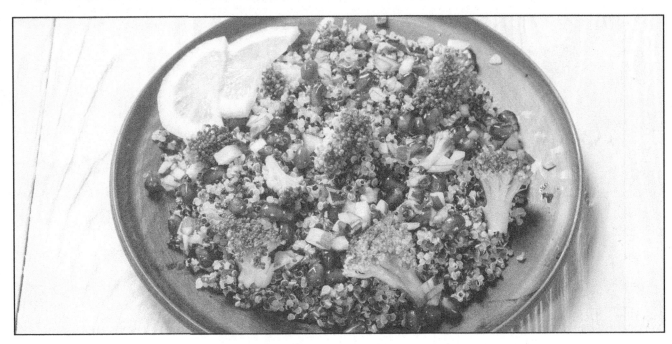

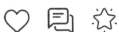

PREPARATION TIME: 5 minutes
COOKING TIME: 10 minutes
SERVINGS: 4
INGREDIENTS:

- 2 Tbsp olive oil
- 1 cup baby potatoes, cut in half
- 1 cup broccoli florets
- 2 cups cooked quinoa
- 1 lemon Zest
- Sea salt and freshly ground pepper, to taste

DIRECTIONS:

1. Heat the olive oil in a large skillet over medium heat until shimmering.
2. Add the potatoes and cook for about 6 to 7 minutes or until softened and golden brown. Add the broccoli and cook for about 3 minutes or until tender.
3. Remove from the heat and add the quinoa and lemon zest. Season with salt and pepper to taste, then serve.

NUTRITION: Calories: 230; Carbs: 39.7 g; Protein: 6.2 g; Fat: 5.3 g.

43. Beet and Bean Burgers

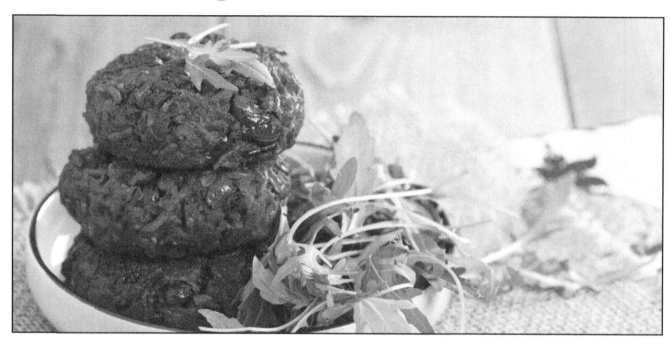

PREPARATION TIME: 15 minutes
COOKING TIME: 35 minutes
SERVINGS: 4
INGREDIENTS:

- 1 Tbsp ginger
- 1 cup gluten-free rolled oats
- 3 cups cooked navy beans (1½ cups dried)
- 2 cups yam/sweet potato purée (about 2 yams/sweet potatoes, steamed and mashed)
- ½ cup sunflower seed butter or tahini
- 1 beet
- ½ tsp salt

DIRECTIONS:

1. Pulse the oats a few times in a food processor until a rough meal forms. Combine the beans, yam purée, sunflower seed butter, beet, ginger and salt in a large mixing bowl. Blend until well combined. You may smooth it out entirely or leave it somewhat lumpy. Refrigerate for 30 minutes to firm up the mixture.
2. Preheat the oven to 350°F. Use parchment paper or Silpat to line a baking sheet. Scoop the mixture onto the prepared sheet using a 13-cup or 12-cup measuring. (The scoop size is determined by the size of the burgers you desire.)
3. Gently pat the ingredients down to make 1-inch thick patties. This recipe makes around 12 patties. Preheat the oven to 350°F and bake the sheet for 35 minutes. Halfway through the cooking period, flip the burgers.

NUTRITION: Calories: 301; Carbs: 40.4 g; Protein: 13.6 g; Fat: 9.2 g.

44. Grilled Mackerel with Asparagus

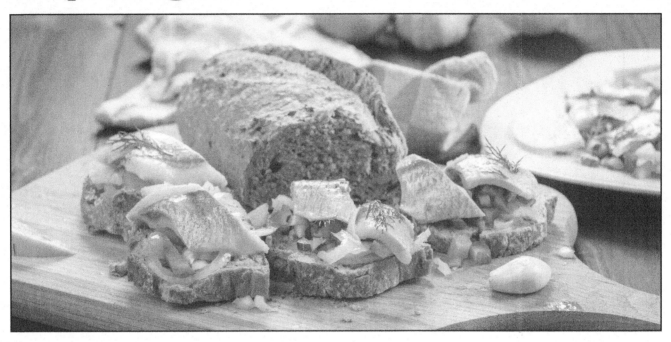

 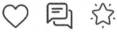

PREPARATION TIME: 10 minutes
COOKING TIME: 5 minutes
SERVINGS: 4
INGREDIENTS:

- 4 slices dark rye bread
- 2 tsp Dijon mustard
- 1 cup packed baby spinach
- 12 thin slices cucumber
- 1 cup packed asparagus
- 1 Tbsp chopped scallions
- 6 oz grilled mackerel
- ¼ tsp salt (optional)
- ¼ tsp freshly ground black pepper (optional)

DIRECTIONS:

1. Toast the bread.
2. Spread each toasted slice with the mustard.
3. Arrange baby spinach over the bread and top with cucumber slices, asparagus and scallions.
4. Divide the mackerel among the four slices of bread. Sprinkle with salt and pepper (if using), and serve.
5. 5If you can't find smoked mackerel, you can substitute smoked salmon or trout or use good-quality canned tuna instead.

NUTRITION: Calories: 197; Carbs: 29.3 g; Protein: 11.5 g; Fat: 3.8 g.

45. Tempeh with Olives and Capers

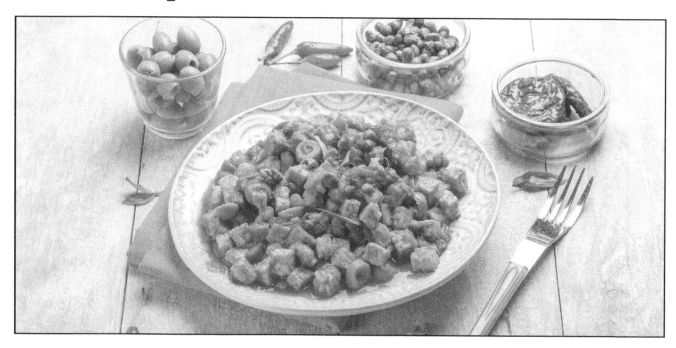

PREPARATION TIME: 5 minutes
COOKING TIME: 8 minutes
SERVINGS: 3
INGREDIENTS:

- 1 lb tempeh
- 2 Tbsp black olives
- 2 chopped shallots
- 2 tsp paprika
- 2 Tbsp olive oil
- 1 pinch salt

DIRECTIONS:

1. In a non-stick pan, lightly heat the olive oil and brown the shallots for 5 minutes. Add the diced tempeh, paprika and chopped olives.
2. Add the salt and pepper, and cook for 3 minutes, stirring.

NUTRITION: Calories: 251; Carbs: 11.3 g; Protein: 20.4 g; Fat: 13.8 g.

46. Rolls of Quinoa Lettuce and Raspberries

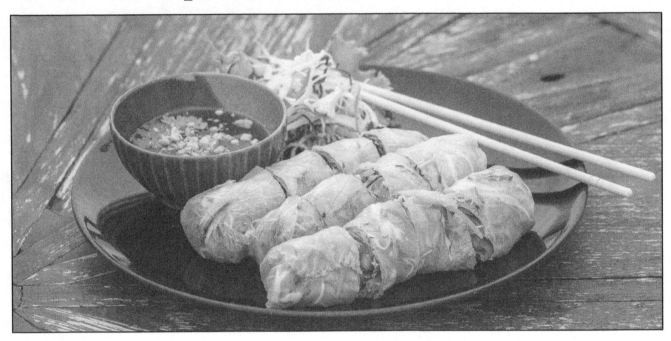

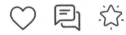

PREPARATION TIME: 15 minutes
COOKING TIME: 15 minutes
SERVINGS: 3
INGREDIENTS:
- 1 cup quinoa
- 1 head lettuce
- 1 cucumber
- 10 cherry tomatoes
- 1 Tbsp chopped fresh mint leaves
- 2 Tbsp raspberries
- 1 organic lemon
- 3 Tbsp olive oil
- 3 Tbsp cottage cheese

DIRECTIONS:
1. Cook the quinoa in plenty of lightly salted water for about 15 minutes, and drain well.
2. Remove the larger leaves from the lettuce without breaking them and wash them. Peel the cucumber and cut it into thin slices. Wash the cherry tomatoes and cut them into four parts.
3. Put the raspberries in a blender with the mint, lemon juice and olive oil, and blend well. Mix the quinoa with the cucumber, cherry tomatoes, cheese and raspberry sauce.
4. Spread the quinoa filling in the center of the salad leaves, and close with a toothpick.

NUTRITION: Calories: 370; Carbs: 44.2 g; Protein: 14.7 g; Fat: 15.1 g.

47. Oven Roasted Root Vegetables with Honey

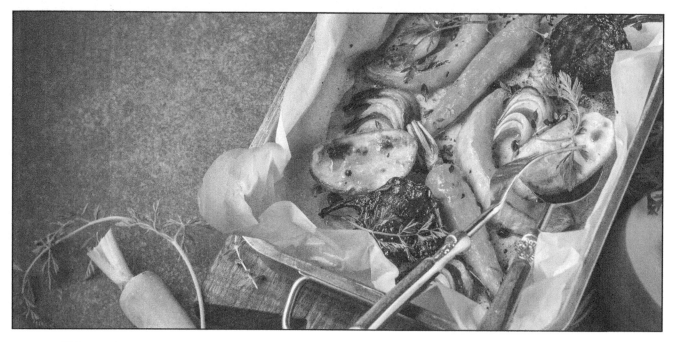

 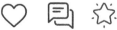

PREPARATION TIME: 15 minutes
COOKING TIME: 25-35 minutes
SERVINGS: 4-6
INGREDIENTS:

- ¼ cup coconut oil, melted
- 1 Tbsp extra-virgin olive oil
- 2 small sweet potatoes, peeled and cut into 1-inch cubes
- 1 bunch beets, peeled and cut into 1-inch cubes
- 4 carrots, peeled and cut into 1-inch rounds
- 3 parsnips, peeled and cut into 1-inch rounds
- 1 Tbsp raw honey or maple syrup
- 1 tsp salt
- ½ tsp freshly ground black pepper

DIRECTIONS:

1. Preheat the oven to 400°F (205°C).
2. Use parchment paper to line 2 rimmed baking sheets.
3. Add the sweet potatoes, beets, carrots and parsnips into a large bowl, and mix until combined. Then mix in the coconut oil, olive oil, honey, salt and pepper. Toss to coat the vegetables.
4. Evenly divide the vegetables between the two baking sheets, spreading them into a single layer.
5. 5. Put the sheets in the preheated oven and bake the vegetables for 10 to 15 minutes. Turn them over and let them brown on the other side. Continue to bake the vegetables for another 10 to 15 minutes or until brown and tender. Serve warm or at room temperature.

NUTRITION: Calories: 251; Carbs: 11.3 g; Protein: 20.4 g; Fat: 13.8 g.

80

48. Red Lentils with Spinach

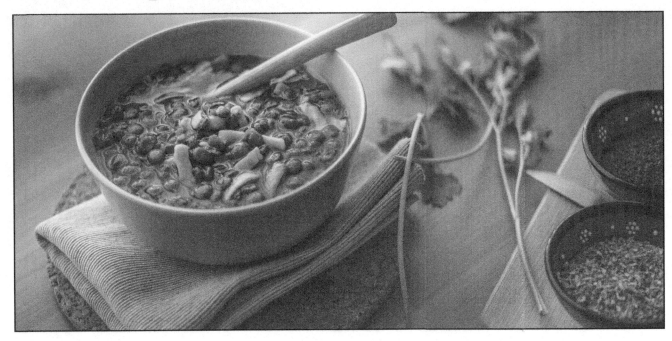

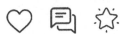 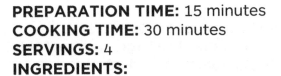

PREPARATION TIME: 15 minutes
COOKING TIME: 30 minutes
SERVINGS: 4
INGREDIENTS:

- 3 ½ cups water
- 1 ½ cups red lentils, soaked for 20 minutes and drained
- ½ tsp red chili powder
- ½ tsp ground turmeric
- Salt, to taste
- 1 lb fresh spinach, chopped
- 2 Tbsp coconut oil
- 1 onion, chopped
- 1 tsp mustard seeds
- 1 tsp ground cumin
- ½ cup coconut milk
- 1 tsp garam masala

DIRECTIONS:

1. Add water, lentils, red chili powder, turmeric and salt in a large pan, and bring to a boil on high heat.
2. Reduce the heat to low and simmer, covered for about 15 minutes.
3. Stir in spinach and simmer for about 5 minutes.
4. In a frying pan, melt coconut oil on medium heat.
5. Add onion, mustard seeds and cumin, and sauté for about 4–5 minutes.
6. Transfer the onion mixture to the pan with the lentils and stir to combine.
7. Stir in coconut milk and garam masala, and simmer for about 3–4 minutes.
8. Serve hot

NUTRITION: Calories: 233; Carbs: 24.8 g; Protein: 12.3 g; Fat: 9.5 g.

49. Broccoli and Cheese Casserole

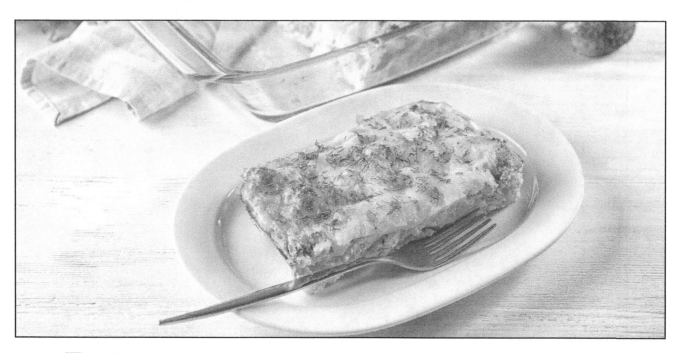

 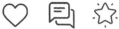

PREPARATION TIME: 10 minutes
COOKING TIME: 35 to 40 minutes
SERVINGS: 2
INGREDIENTS:

- 2 broccoli heads, crowns and stalks finely chopped
- 2 cups cooked pinto or navy beans, or 1 (14-oz, 397 g) can
- 1 to 2 Tbsp Brown rice flour or arrowroot flour
- 1 tsp Salt
- 2 tsp cheese
- ¾ cup vegetable broth or water
- ½ cup walnuts, chopped

DIRECTIONS:

1. Preheat the oven to 350°F(180°C).
2. Add the broth into a large ovenproof pot, warming over medium heat.
3. Mix in the broccoli and salt. Cook for 6 to 8 minutes until the broccoli is bright green.
4. Add the pinto beans, cheese and brown rice flour. Cook for 5 minutes more or until the liquid thickens slightly, stirring often.
5. Sprinkle the top with the walnuts.
6. Transfer the pot to the preheated oven and bake for 20 to 25 minutes. The walnuts should be toasted. Remove from the oven and serve hot.

NUTRITION: Calories: 428; Carbs: 51.3 g; Protein: 31.1 g; Fat: 11.2 g.

50. Baked Potatoes Stuffed With Vegetables

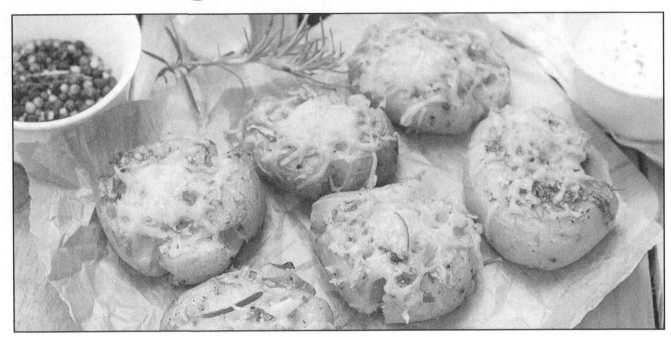

 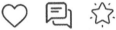

PREPARATION TIME: 15 minutes
COOKING TIME: 90 minutes
SERVINGS: 2
INGREDIENTS:

- 1 tsp olive oil
- ¼ cup Cheddar cheese shredded
- 1 medium-sized baking potato
- ½ tsp salt
- 1 pinch black pepper freshly ground
- 2 tsp butter

DIRECTIONS:

1. Preheat oven to 300◻. Scrub the potato and penetrate the skin with a fork or knife numerous times.
2. Apply olive oil to the skin before applying salt. Bake for about 90 minutes, just until the potato is somewhat tender and nicely browned, in a preheated oven.
3. Serve the potato using butter and black pepper, sliced along the middle. If desired, grate some grated Cheddar cheese on top.

NUTRITION: Calories: 420; Carbs: 38.6 g; Protein: 13.2 g; Fat: 23.4 g.

51. Green Curry

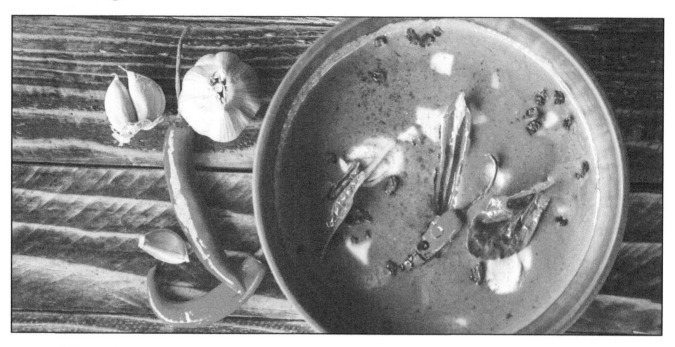

PREPARATION TIME: 10 minutes
COOKING TIME: 30 minutes
SERVINGS: 2
INGREDIENTS:
- 2 Tbsp extra-virgin olive oil
- 2 garlic cloves, minced
- 1 onion, chopped
- 1 Tbsp grated ginger
- 1 Tbsp green curry paste
- 4 cups vegetable broth
- 1 lb butternut squash, cubed
- Sea salt and pepper, to taste
- ¼ cup coconut milk
- 2 Tbsp cilantro, minced

DIRECTIONS:
1. Warm the olive oil in a pot over medium heat. Place the onion, garlic and ginger, and soften for 5 minutes.
2. Add vegetable broth, butternut squash, green curry paste, salt and pepper, and simmer for 10–15 minutes until the squash is soft.
3. Add coconut milk and purée with a stick blender. Garnish with cilantro.
4. 4. Serve warm.

NUTRITION: Calories: 247; Carbs: 13.9 g; Protein: 5.5 g; Fat: 19.0 g.

52. Shrimp in Curry Sauce

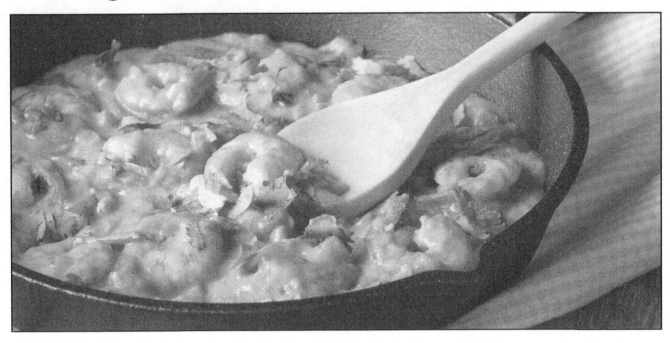

 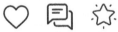

PREPARATION TIME: 5 minutes
COOKING TIME: 10 minutes
SERVINGS: 4
INGREDIENTS:
- 1 sliced onion
- 3 Tbsp olive oil
- 2 tsp curry powder
- 1 cup coconut milk
- 1 cauliflower
- 1 lb Shrimp tails

DIRECTIONS:
1. Add the onion to your oil.
2. Sauté to make it a bit soft.
3. Steam your vegetables in the meantime.
4. Add the curry seasoning, coconut milk and spices if you want once the onion has become soft.
5. Cook for 2 minutes.
6. Include the shrimp. Cook for 5 minutes.
7. Serve with steamed vegetables.

NUTRITION: Calories: 229; Carbs: 4.2 g; Protein: 15.1 g; Fat: 16.8 g.

53. Roasted Broccoli and Ham Casserole

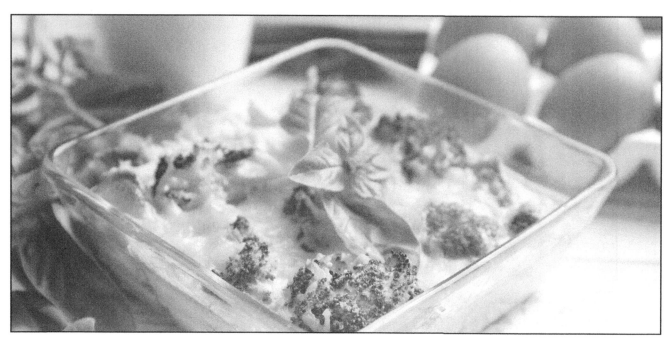

 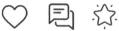

PREPARATION TIME: 15 minutes
COOKING TIME: 30 minutes
SERVINGS: 4
INGREDIENTS:
- 1 head broccoli, florets only, cut into bite-sized pieces
- 2 Tbsp olive oil
- Salt and pepper, to taste
- 1 cup cooked ham, cubed
- ½ cup Parmesan or Romana cheese, grated
- 1 red bell pepper, finely chopped
- 3 scallions, chopped
- 12 eggs
- 2 tsp herbes de Provence

DIRECTIONS:
1. Preheat the oven to 425°F and pre-pare a 9x13" casserole dish with cooking spray.
2. In a large bowl, combine the broccoli with the olive oil, salt and pepper; transfer to a baking sheet.
3. Roast for 25 minutes until browned, then remove the pan from the oven. Reduce the oven temperature to 375°F.
4. Gently combine the roasted broccoli, ham, Parmesan, red bell pepper and scallions in a large bowl. Move the mixture to the prepared baking dish.
5. In a large mixing bowl, lightly beat the eggs and stir in the herbes de Provence. With salt and pepper, season it. Pour over the broccoli mixture.
6. Bake for 35 minutes until the surface is lightly browned and the eggs are cooked.

NUTRITION: Calories: 350; Carbs: 5.2 g; Protein: 32.6 g; Fat: 22.3 g. .

54. Italian Eggplant Casserole

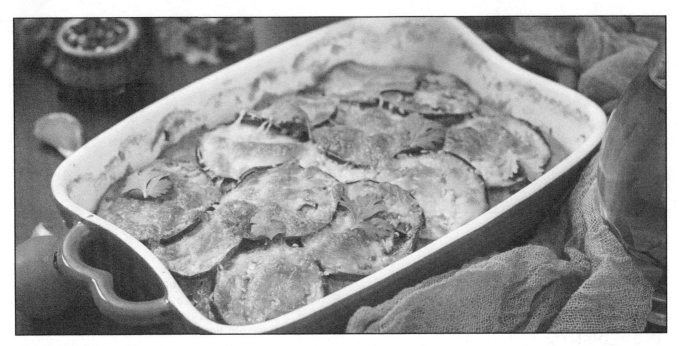

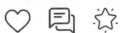

PREPARATION TIME: 20 minutes
COOKING TIME: 40 minutes
SERVINGS: 4
INGREDIENTS:

- 1 (1 lb) eggplant, peeled, cubed
- ½ cup seasoned bread crumbs, divided
- ½ cup liquid egg substitute
- ½ tsp Garlic powder
- ¼ tsp Italian seasoning
- ⅛ tsp Black pepper
- ⅛ tsp salt
- 2 tomatoes, sliced

DIRECTIONS:

1. Bring 2 inches of water to a boil in a soup pot. Add the eggplant, cover, and simmer for 20 to 30 minutes until tender. Drain.
2. Set the oven to 350°F. Spray cooking spray in a 9-inch square baking dish.
3. With a fork, mash the eggplant in a medium basin. Add the egg substitute, Italian seasoning, garlic, salt, pepper and ¼ cup of bread crumbs.
4. Slices of tomato should be placed on the spread eggplant mixture in the baking dish. Cooking spray is applied to the tomatoes before the remaining bread crumbs are added.
5. Bake for 25 to 30 minutes or until the tomatoes are soft and the edges are browned

NUTRITION: Calories: 132; Carbs: 19.3 g; Protein: 8.3 g; Fat: 2.5 g.

55. Butternut Squash Casserole

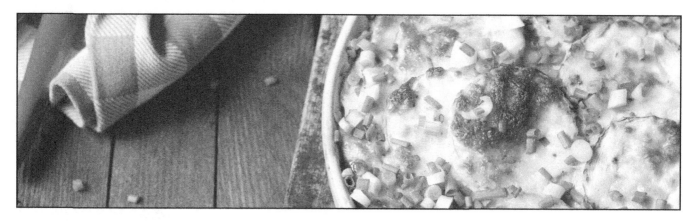

PREPARATION TIME: 15 minutes
COOKING TIME: 30 minutes
SERVINGS: 4
INGREDIENTS:
- 1 Tbsp olive oil
- 2 cups chopped onion
- 10 cup baby spinach
- ¾ cup sharp provolone cheese, shredded
- ½ cup chopped fresh flat-leaf parsley
- 1 tsp salt
- ½ tsp black pepper
- 1 tsp oregano
- 2 large eggs
- 2 (15 oz) containers 2% cottage cheese
- 3 cup butternut squash, peeled and diced
- 6 cups marinara or pasta sauce
- 12 oven-ready lasagna noodles (no boiling)
- 1 cup fresh Parmesan cheese, grated

DIRECTIONS:
1. Preheat the oven to 375°F. Coat the bottom and sides of two 8x8" baking dishes with cooking spray.
2. Heat a large Dutch oven over medium-high heat. Add the oil and onion; sauté 4 minutes or until tender.
3. Add the spinach and stir until the spinach wilts. Remove the pot from the heat. In a large bowl, combine the provolone, parsley, salt, pepper, oregano, eggs and cottage cheese.
4. Put the squash in a microwave-safe basin for 5 minutes, with the lid on, or until tender.
5. In each baking dish, carry out the following actions: Pasta sauce or marinara sauce should cover the bottom of the dish by half a cup. Spread 1 cup of the cheese mixture over the noodles after placing 2 on top of the sauce. Place 1 ½ cups squash cubes and ¾ cup sauce on the cheese mixture.
6. Spread 1 cup of the cheese mixture over the noodles after placing 2 on top of the sauce. Spread ¾ cup of sauce over the cheese mixture after adding 1 ½ cups of the onion mixture.
7. Place 2 noodles over the sauce, then equally distribute 1 cup of marinara over the noodles. Add ½ cup of Parmesan cheese.
8. Wrap foil around each pan. After the first 30 minutes of baking, remove the foil and bake for 30 minutes.
9. 9. To freeze unbaked lasagna: Prepare through step 8. Cover with plastic wrap, pressing to remove as much air as possible. Wrap with heavy-duty foil. Store in the freezer for up to 2 months.
10. 10. To prepare frozen unbaked lasagna: Thaw completely in the refrigerator (about 24 hours). Preheat the oven to 375°F. Remove the foil and set it aside. Discard the plastic wrap. Cover the lasagna with the reserved foil; bake at 375° for 1 hour. Uncover and bake for an additional 30 minutes or until bubbly.

NUTRITION: Calories: 350; Carbs: 5.2 g; Protein: 32.6 g; Fat: 22.3 g. .

56. Eggplant Parmesan Casserole

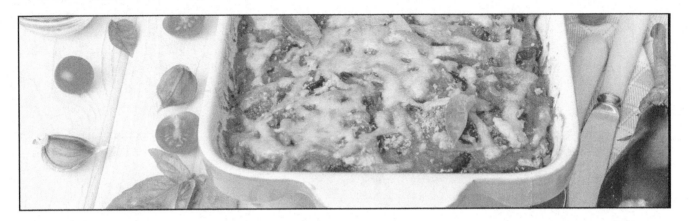

PREPARATION TIME: 10 minutes
COOKING TIME: 60 minutes
SERVINGS: 4
INGREDIENTS:

- 2 large eggs, lightly beaten
- 1 Tbsp water
- 2 cups panko breadcrumbs
- ¼ cup Parmigiano-Reggiano cheese, grated
- 2 (1 lb) eggplants, peeled and cut croswise into ½-inch slices

For the Filling:
- ½ cup fresh basil, chopped
- ¼ cup Parmigiano-Reggiano cheese, grated
- ½ tsp crushed red pepper
- 3 garlic cloves, minced
- 1 tsp onion powder
- Salt and pepper, to taste
- 2 (8 oz) containers of 2% cottage cheese
- 1 large egg, lightly beaten

For the Topping:
- 4 cup pasta sauce
- 1 ½ cup mozzarella cheese, shredded

DIRECTIONS:
1. A 9x13" baking dish and 2 cookie sheets should be prepared with cooking spray and placed in the preheated 375°F oven.
2. Get the eggplant ready. In a small dish, mix the eggs with 1 Tbsp of water. In a second shallow dish, combine the panko and ¼ cup of Parmigiano-Reggiano.
3. Each slice of eggplant is first dipped in the egg mixture, then gently pressed into the panko mixture so the breadcrumbs adhere and any excess is shaken off.
4. On the baking sheets, space the greased eggplant slices 1 inch apart. They should be baked for 30 minutes, turning them once and rotating the oven sheets after 15 minutes or until they are brown.
5. The basil, ¼ cup of Parmigiano-Reggiano cheese, garlic, onion powder, salt, pepper, cottage cheese and egg go into the filling's preparation.
6. Pour 12 cups of spaghetti sauce into the baking dish to assemble. Over the pasta sauce, arrange half of the eggplant slices.
7. Spread half of the cottage cheese mixture over the sauce, then top with approximately ¾ cup of pasta sauce. Add a third of the mozzarella next. Once more, layer the ingredients, finishing with roughly a cup of pasta sauce.
8. Cooking spray-coated aluminum foil should be used to cover tightly — 35 minutes at 375 °F baking. Add the final third of the mozzarella and take off the foil.
9. Bake for 10 minutes or until the cheese has melted and the sauce is bubbling; let it cool before serving.

NUTRITION: Calories: 335; Carbs: 24.3 g; Protein: 23.5 g; Fat: 16.0 g.

57. Pumpkin Pie

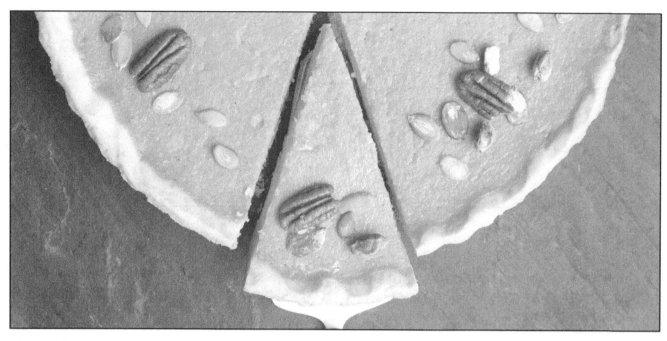

 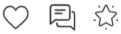

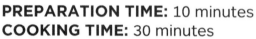

PREPARATION TIME: 10 minutes
COOKING TIME: 30 minutes
SERVINGS: 3
INGREDIENTS:
- ½ cup flaked coconut
- ½ cup sunflower seeds
- ¼ cup sliced almonds
- 2/3 cup almond flour
- 1 egg
- ¼ cup pumpkin puree
- ¼ cup coconut oil
- 1 ½ tsp baking powder
- ¼ cup erythritol
- 2/3 tsp pumpkin pie spice
- ¼ tsp salt
- ½ tsp vanilla extract

DIRECTIONS:
1. Preheat the oven to 325°F.
2. Process sunflower seeds and coconut oil in a blender. Mix the rest of the ingredients in another bowl and add the prepared puree.
3. Spread on the pan and bake for around 20 minutes.

NUTRITION: Calories: 224; Carbs: 10.8 g; Protein: 6.5 g; Fat: 17.3 g.

58. Carrot Cookies with Dark Chocolate

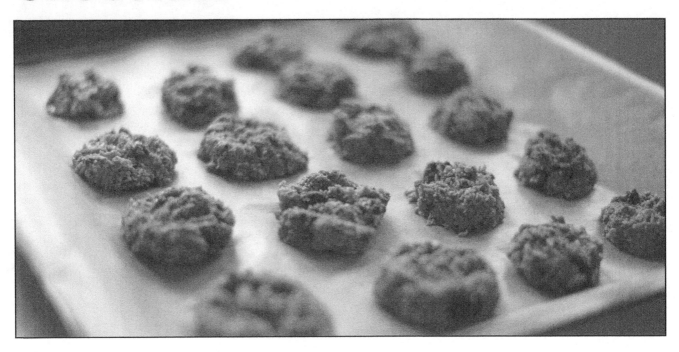

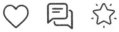

PREPARATION TIME: 15 minutes
COOKING TIME: 20 minutes
SERVINGS:15
INGREDIENTS:

- 1 cup oats
- ¼ cup honey
- 1 cup whole flour
- 2 tsp cinnamon
- 1 tsp ginger
- ½ tsp baking powder
- 1 cup grated carrots
- 2 tsp dark chocolate
- 1 tsp nutmeg
- ½ cup avocado or olive oil
- 1 large orange

DIRECTIONS:

1. Preheat the oven to 350°F and prepare a baking sheet and parchment paper. Combine the flour, oats, cinnamon, ginger, nutmeg, and baking powder in a large mixing basin.
2. Mix the carrots, oil and honey until everything is well blended. Combine the orange zest and the other ingredients in a mixing bowl. Scoop rounded Tbsp of batter onto the baking sheet that has been prepared.
3. Flatten the cookies to a thickness of approximately 12 inches. Bake for 15 to 20 minutes until cooked through and gently browned on the bottoms.
4. Allow it to rest for a few minutes before transferring it to a wire rack to cool. Warm or at room temperature is OK.
5. The cookies may be refrigerated for up to 5 days or frozen for 6 months in an airtight container.

NUTRITION: Calories: 114; Carbs: 16.0 g; Protein: 2.7 g; Fat: 4.3 g.

91

59. Quinoa and Chocolate Cake

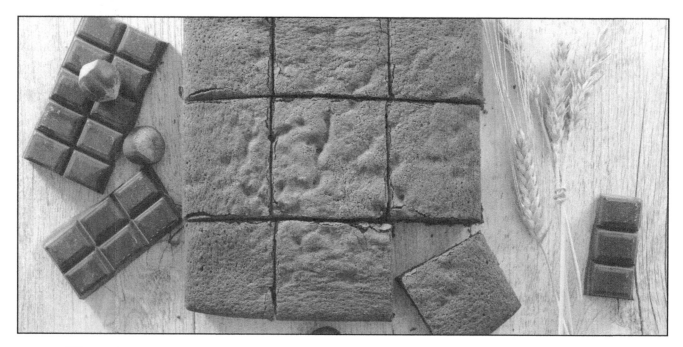

 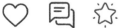

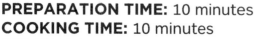

PREPARATION TIME: 10 minutes
COOKING TIME: 10 minutes
SERVINGS: 18
INGREDIENTS:

- 2 eggs (lightly beaten)
- 1 ½ cups almond flour
- 3 Tbsp butter
- 3 Tbsp quinoa
- 3 Tbsp unsweetened cocoa powder
- 1 tsp vanilla
- ¼ cup Swerve
- 3 oz Unsweetened chocolate (chopped)
- Pinch salt

DIRECTIONS:

1. Melt the chocolate, butter, quinoa and cocoa powder in a saucepan over low heat.
2. Remove the pan from the heat and put it aside. Whisk the eggs, vanilla and salt, and swerve in a mixing bowl until thoroughly blended.
3. Mix the melted chocolate mixture thoroughly into the egg mixture. Mix in the almond flour until everything is nicely mixed. Set aside for 1 hour in the refrigerator.
4. Preheat the oven to 325°F. Spray a baking pan with cooking spray and line it with parchment paper. Bake for 10 minutes after scooping out the mixture onto a baking pan.
5. Serve and have fun.

NUTRITION: Calories: 64; Carbs: 4.9 g; Protein: 2.0 g; Fat: 3.8 g.

60. Lemon Semi-Integral Flour Plum Cake

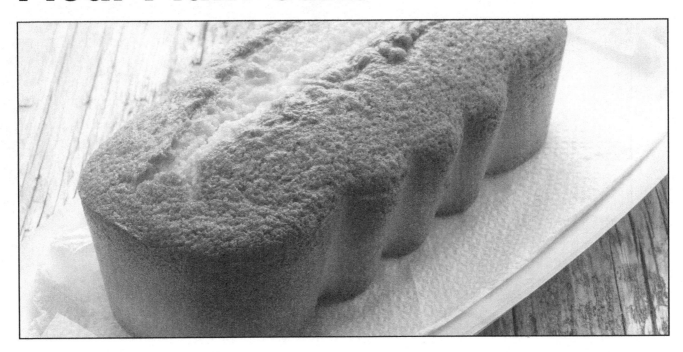

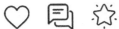

PREPARATION TIME: 10 minutes
COOKING TIME: 40 minutes
SERVINGS: 4
INGREDIENTS:

- 7 oz almond flour
- 1 egg, whisked
- 5 Tbsp Stevia
- 3 oz warm almond milk
- 2 lb plums, pitted and cut into quarters
- 2 apples, cored and chopped
- 1 lemon Zest, grated
- 1 tsp baking powder

DIRECTIONS:

1. In a bowl, mix the almond milk with the egg, stevia and the rest of the ingredients except the cooking spray and whisk well.
2. Grease a cake pan with the oil, pour the cake mix inside, introduce it into the oven, and bake at 350° F for 40 minutes.
3. Cool down, slice, and serve.

NUTRITION: Calories: 355; Carbs: 41.3 g; Protein: 9.8 g; Fat: 16.8 g.

61. Anti-inflammatory Lemon Bars

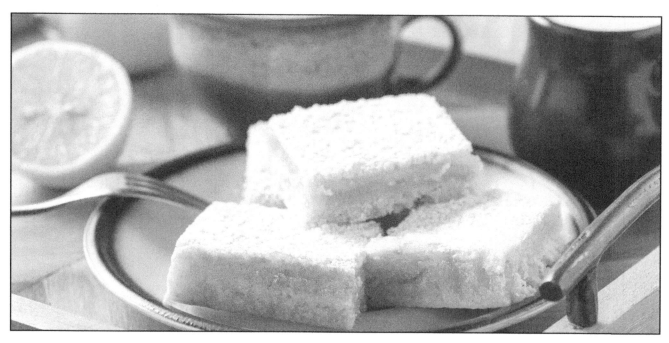

 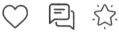

PREPARATION TIME: 15 minutes
COOKING TIME: 30 minutes
SERVINGS: 5
INGREDIENTS:

- 1 cup almond flour
- ½ cup lemon juice
- ½ cup coconut flour
- 1 tsp baking soda
- 2 Tbsp honey
- 2 Tbsp cashew butter
- 2 Tbsp lemon zest
- 1 tsp ground ginger

DIRECTIONS:

1. In a mixing bowl, combine the almond flour, coconut flour, baking soda, lemon zest and ground ginger together. Stir the mixture gently.
2. Add the honey, cashew butter and lemon juice.
3. Knead into a soft dough.
4. Roll the dough with a rolling pin.
5. Transfer the dough to a tray and cover it with baking paper.
6. Preheat the oven to 350°F and place the tray in the oven.
7. Cook the dish for 30 minutes.
8. Remove the cooked dish from the oven and cut it into bars.
9. Cool the bars slightly and serve them immediately.

NUTRITION: Calories: 350; Carbs: 5.2 g; Protein: 32.6 g; Fat: 22.3 g.

62. Chocolate Muffins

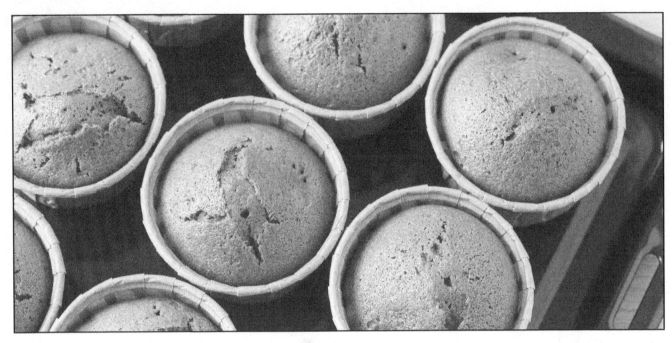

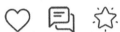

PREPARATION TIME: 20 minutes
COOKING TIME: 20 minutes
SERVINGS: 5
INGREDIENTS:

- 2 cups coconut flour
- 1 tsp baking powder
- 1 Tbsp apple cider vinegar
- 1 tsp salt
- 3 Tbsp honey
- 1 Tbsp raw cocoa powder
- 2 Tbsp cashew butter
- ½ cup almond milk, unsweetened
- 2 Tbsp lemon juice
- 1 Tbsp olive oil

DIRECTIONS:

1. Place the coconut flour in the mixing bowl and add baking powder.
2. Add the cocoa powder and salt, and mix
3. In a separate bowl, combine the apple cider vinegar, honey, cashew butter, almond milk, lemon juice and olive oil. Whisk the mixture.
4. Pour the liquid mixture into the coconut flour mixture slowly, whisking it constantly.
5. When you get a smooth batter, let it sit for 10 minutes.
6. Meanwhile, preheat the oven to 350°F.
7. Fill muffin molds halfway up with the batter.
8. Transfer the muffins to the preheated oven.
9. Cook the muffins for 20 minutes.
10. When the muffins are cooked, remove them from the oven and cool them well.
11. Then remove the muffins from the molds
12. Serve the dish immediately

NUTRITION: Calories: 255; Carbs: 12.3 g; Protein: 6.4 g; Fat: 18.8 g.

63. Poppy Seed Cake

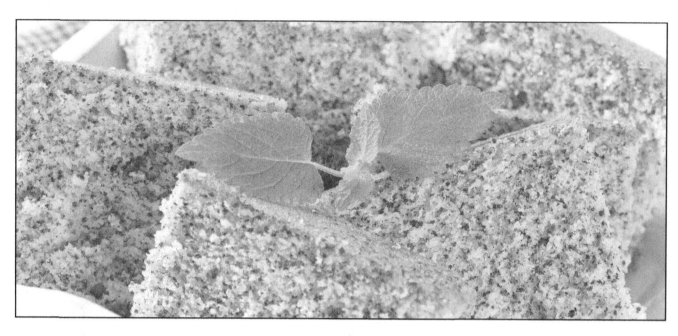

PREPARATION TIME: 15 minutes
COOKING TIME: 40 minutes
SERVINGS: 6
INGREDIENTS:
- 1 cup arrowroot flour
- 2 cups almond flour
- ½ cup almond slices
- 3 oz poppy seeds
- 1 tsp vanilla extract
- 1 tsp cinnamon
- 1 tsp nutmeg
- 1 tsp baking powder
- 1 Tbsp apple cider vinegar
- 1 cup coconut milk, unsweetened
- 3 Tbsp liquid stevia
- 1 tsp lime zest
- 3 Tbsp cashew butter

DIRECTIONS:
1. Combine the arrowroot flour and almond flour together.
2. Add the almond slices and poppy seeds.
3. Add the cinnamon, nutmeg, baking soda and lime zest.
4. Mix well.
5. Add the liquid ingredients, beginning with the vanilla extract, apple cider vinegar and coconut milk.
6. Then add liquid stevia and cashew butter.
7. Mix and knead the smooth dough.
8. Preheat the oven to 350°F.
9. Cover a tray with baking paper.
10. Transfer the dough to the tray.
11. Cover the dough with the parchment and transfer it into the oven.
12. Cook the cake for 40 minutes.
13. Remove the cake from the oven and chill it well.
14. Remove the cake from the tray and slice it.
15. 15. Serve the cake.
16.

NUTRITION: Calories: 376; Carbs: 24.2 g; Protein: 11.8 g; Fat: 25.8 g.

64. Aromatic Cherry tart

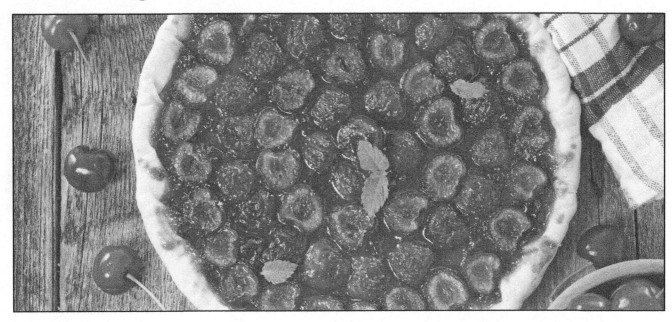

PREPARATION TIME: 15 minutes
COOKING TIME: 40 minutes
SERVINGS: 6
INGREDIENTS:
- 1 cup coconut flour
- 1 cup almond flour
- 1 tsp cinnamon
- 1 tsp anise
- 3 Tbsp honey
- 1 cup cherries, pitted
- 6 Tbsp cashew butter
- ¼ cup coconut milk, unsweetened
- 1 tsp vanilla extract
- 1 tsp baking soda
- 3 Tbsp lemon juice
- 1 tsp mint

DIRECTIONS:
1. Place the coconut flour and almond flour in the mixing bowl.
2. Add cinnamon and anise. Stir the mixture gently.
3. Add the cashew butter, coconut milk, baking soda, lemon juice and mint.
4. Knead into a smooth and pliable dough.
5. Chop the cherries and combine them with vanilla extract and honey.
6. Mix well.
7. Roll the dough with a rolling pin.
8. Place the dough on a tray.
9. Sprinkle the dough with the chopped cherry mixture.
10. Preheat the oven to 350°F and transfer the tart into the oven.
11. Cook the tart for 30 minutes or until it is done.
12. Remove the tart from the oven and chill it well.
13. 13. Slice it and serve.
14. 14. Enjoy!

NUTRITION: Calories: 373; Carbs: 18.3 g; Protein: 11.2 g; Fat: 28.3 g.

65. Baked Sweet Potato Chips

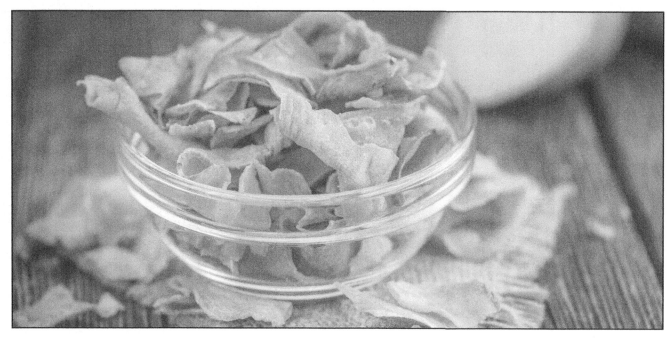

 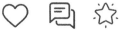   ●

PREPARATION TIME: 20 minutes
COOKING TIME: 2 hours
SERVINGS: 2
INGREDIENTS:
- 2 large sweet potatoes, sliced as thin as possible
- 3 Tbsp Extra-virgin olive oil
- 1 tsp Sea salt

DIRECTIONS:
1. Preheat the oven to 250°F(120°C).
2. Set the rack in the center of the oven.
3. Add the sweet potato slices and the olive oil into a large bowl, tossing them together. Arrange the slices in a single layer on two baking sheets. Sprinkle with sea salt.
4. Put the sheets in the preheated oven and bake for about 2 hours; after baking for 1 hour, rotate the pans and flip the chips, then bake the remaining 1 hour.
5. Bake until the chips are lightly brown and crisp, remove them from the oven. Some may be a bit soft, but they will crisp as they cool. Cool the chips for 10 minutes before serving.
6. 6. Serve immediately. Cause the chips to lose their crunch within several hours.

NUTRITION: Calories: 350; Carbs: 5.2 g; Protein: 32.6 g; Fat: 22.3 g. .

66. Dried Banana Chips

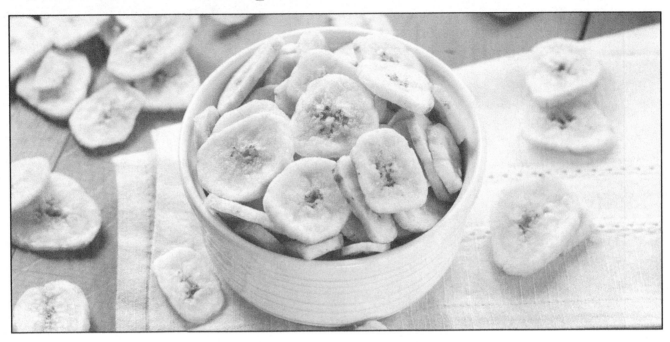

 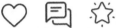

PREPARATION TIME: 10 minutes
COOKING TIME: 20 minutes
SERVINGS: 2
INGREDIENTS:

- ¼ cup olive oil
- 2 lb plantains, peeled and sliced thinly on the diagonal
- ½ tsp Kosher salt
- ½ tsp Smoked paprika

DIRECTIONS:

1. Preheat the oven to 375°F (190°C). Use parchment paper to line two baking sheets.
2. On the prepared baking sheets, lay the plantain slices in a single layer. Use half of the olive oil to brush the tops of the slices, then turn them over and use oil to brush the other side. Sprinkle with salt and paprika.
3. Roast for 18 to 20 minutes until the plantains are crunchy and golden, turning halfway through. Allow them to cool completely.
4. Transfer into an airtight container and store at room temperature for up to 3 days.

NUTRITION: Calories: 334; Carbs: 37.5 g; Protein: 2.4 g; Fat: 18.6 g.

67. Roasted Chickpeas

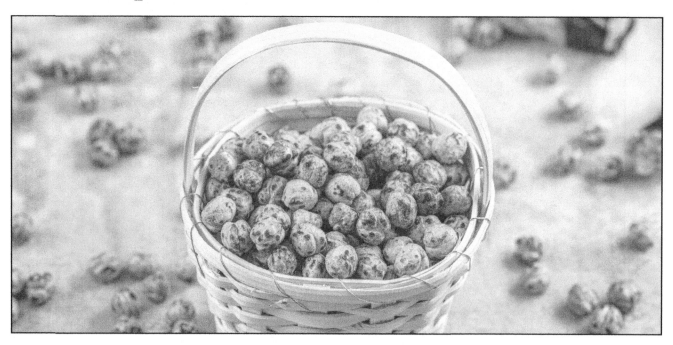

PREPARATION TIME: 5 minutes
COOKING TIME: 1hour 30 minutes
SERVINGS: 8
INGREDIENTS:
- 2 Tbsp extra-virgin olive oil
- 1 cup dried chickpeas, soaked in water for 8 hours
- 1 tsp onion powder, plus additional as needed
- 1 Tbsp garlic powder, plus additional as needed
- ¾ tsp salt, plus additional as needed

DIRECTIONS:
1. Drain and rinse the chickpeas well. In a large pot, cover the chickpeas with a few inches of water. Bring to a boil over medium-high heat. Cook the chickpeas until tender, about 45 minutes. Drain well.
2. Preheat the oven to 325°F(165°C).
3. Use aluminum foil to line a large baking sheet.
4. Add the chickpeas, olive oil, garlic powder, onion powder and salt to a large bowl, tossing them together.
5. Taste the mixture and adjust the seasoning if needed. The flavors intensify as the chickpeas bake.
6. On the prepared sheet, spread the chickpeas. Remember, don't crowd the chickpeas, you may need two sheets.
7. Place the sheet(s) in the preheated oven and bake for about 45 minutes, until golden and crunchy, stirring and turning the chickpeas every 15 minutes. The chickpeas will crisp as they cool.

NUTRITION: Calories: 78; Carbs: 9.4 g; Protein: 4.5 g; Fat: 2.6 g.

68. Superfoods Bars with a Mix of Nuts and Seeds

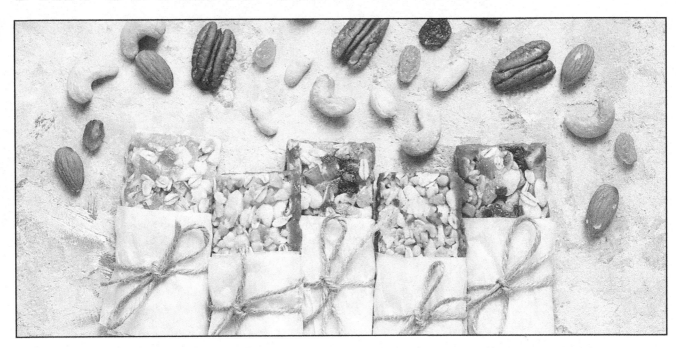

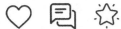

PREPARATION TIME: 10 minutes
COOKING TIME: 15 minutes
SERVINGS: 2
INGREDIENTS:

- 1 cup almonds
- ½ cup walnuts
- ¼ cup sunflower seeds
- ¼ cup pumpkin seeds
- 1 tsp ground turmeric
- ½ tsp ground cumin
- ¼ tsp garlic powder
- ¼ tsp red pepper flakes

DIRECTIONS:

1. Preheat the oven to 350°F (180°c).
2. Add all the ingredients to a bowl, mixing well.
3. Spread the nuts evenly on a rimmed baking sheet, baking until lightly toasted, about 10 to 15 minutes.
4. Set aside until cool completely.
5. Enjoy.

NUTRITION: Calories: 188; Carbs: 4.8 g; Protein: 6.1 g; Fat: 16.2 g.

69. Peanut Butter Protein Bars

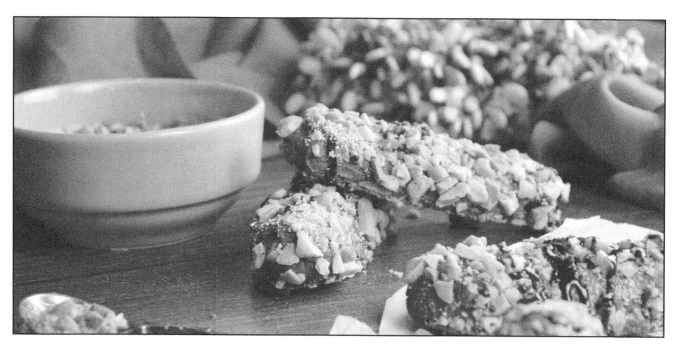

PREPARATION TIME: 10 minutes
COOKING TIME: 10 minutes
SERVINGS: 12
INGREDIENTS:

- 1 cup egg white protein powder
- 2 cups nuts (walnuts, cashews, pecans, or almonds)
- 3 Tbsp instant coffee
- 3 Tbsp peanut butter
- ¼ cup cocoa powder
- 18 dated, pitted

DIRECTIONS:

1. Use parchment paper to line your pan. Set aside.
2. Process the egg white protein, nuts, coffee powder, peanut butter and cocoa powder in a bowl. The nuts should break down into small pieces.
3. Add the pitted dates. Process to combine well.
4. Process until you see the mixture becoming sticky.
5. Stir the cocoa nibs in.
6. Transfer the mixture to your pan. Press into the pan evenly with your hands.
7. Refrigerate for an hour. Cut into squares with a knife.

NUTRITION: Calories: 169; Carbs: 7.5 g; Protein: 13.2 g; Fat: 9.6 g.

70. Beet Chips

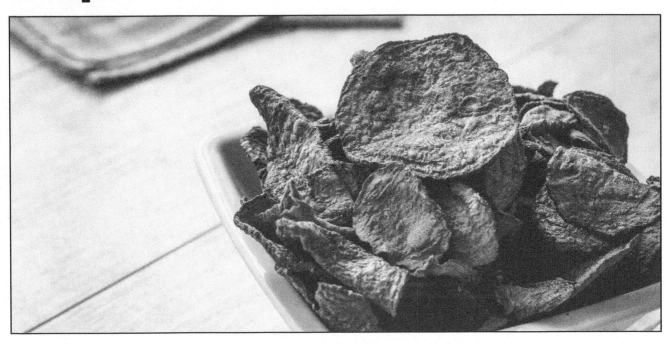

♡ 🗩 ☆   ○ ●

PREPARATION TIME: 10 minutes
COOKING TIME: 30 minutes
SERVINGS: 2
INGREDIENTS:
- 1 beetroot, trimmed, peeled, and thinly sliced
- 1 tsp garlic, minced
- 2 tsp coconut oil, melted

DIRECTIONS:
1. Preheat your oven to 350°F.
2. Line a baking sheet with parchment paper.
3. In a bowl, add beet slices and oil, and toss to coat well.
4. Arrange the beet slices onto the prepared baking sheet in a single layer.
5. Bake for approximately 20–30 minutes.
6. Serve immediately.

NUTRITION: alories: 74; Carbs: 6.1 g; Protein: 1.4 g; Fat: 5.0 g.

71. Butternut Fries

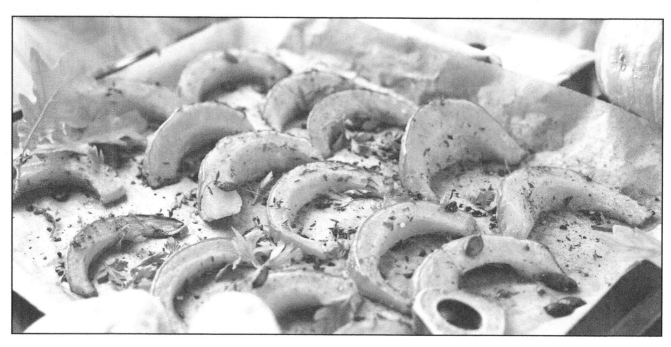

 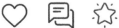

PREPARATION TIME: 20 minutes
COOKING TIME: 45 minutes
SERVINGS: 4
INGREDIENTS:
- ¾ tsp salt
- 2 Tbsp coconut oil
- 1 (large) butternut squash, cut into (3 inches-long and ½ inch-thick) pieces
- 3 sprigs rosemary, chopped

DIRECTIONS:
1. The oven should be set to 375°F.
2. A large baking sheet should be lined with aluminum foil or parchment paper.
3. In a large bowl, combine the salt, squash chunks and coconut oil. Spread the butternut squash over the baking sheet that has been preheated.
4. The baking sheet needs to be baked for 15–20 minutes. Flip the fries over.
5. Add 10 more minutes to the baking time.
6. The fries should be topped with rosemary. Continue baking the fries for another 10–15 minutes or until they reach your desired level of browning. Serve right away.

NUTRITION: Calories: 61; Carbs: 3.8 g; Protein: 0.3 g; Fat: 5.0 g.

72. Date-Ginger Bars

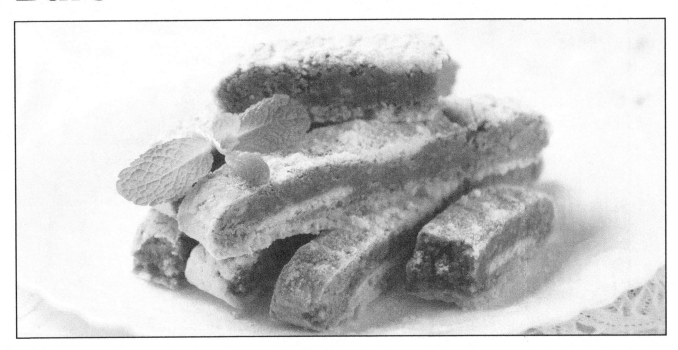

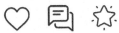

PREPARATION TIME: 10 minutes
COOKING TIME: 20 minutes
SERVINGS: 6
INGREDIENTS:
- ¾ cup dates
- ¼ cup almond milk
- 1 cup almond flour
- 1 tsp ginger, ground

DIRECTIONS:
1. Set the oven to 350°F.
2. In a blender, combine the almond milk and dates. Blend for 5 minutes to produce a paste.
3. In a mixing bowl, combine the ginger and almond flour. Take 3 more minutes of blending.
4. The mixture should come halfway up a baking pan. A 20-minute baking period
5. Give it some time to cool. Make 8 bars out of the cake. Serve.

NUTRITION: Calories: 111; Carbs: 12.4 g; Protein: 3.2 g; Fat: 5.5 g

73. Delicious Zucchini Chips

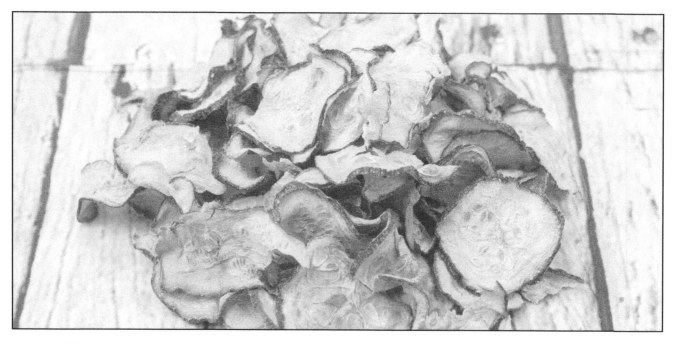

 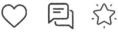

PREPARATION TIME: 15 minutes
COOKING TIME: 2 hours
SERVINGS: 6
INGREDIENTS:
- 2 medium-sized zucchinis, thinly sliced
- 1½ tsp oregano, dried
- 2 Tbsp olive oil, extra-virgin
- ½ tsp salt
- 1½ tsp rosemary, dried
- 1½ tsp basil, dried

DIRECTIONS:
1. Set the oven to the lowest temperature, which is typically between 175 and 200°F.
2. Two baking pans can be lined with parchment paper.
3. Combine the zucchini and olive oil in a sizable mixing bowl.
4. Combine the rosemary, salt, oregano and basil in a small bowl. Sprinkle the zucchini with the herb mixture. Combine everything with your hands, making sure the zucchini is coated evenly.
5. On the baking sheets, organize the zucchini in one layer. They might be very close to one another.
6. Bake the sheets in a preheated oven for 1.5 to 2 hours or until they are dried and crispy. Using the lowest setting on your oven and thinly slicing the zucchini thin will affect how long it takes to bake.
7. Give it time to cool completely. Keep the jar tightly closed.

NUTRITION: Calories: 78; Carbs: 9.4 g; Protein: 4.5 g; Fat: 2.6 g.

74. Roasted Apricots

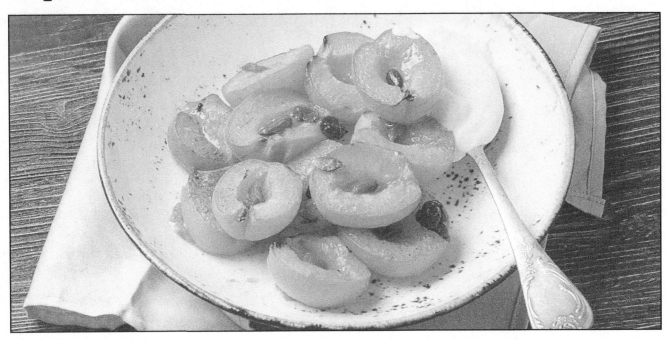

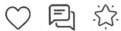

PREPARATION TIME: 10 minutes
COOKING TIME: 30 minutes
SERVINGS: 4
INGREDIENTS:
- 2 Tbsp coconut oil
- 20 apricots, quartered
- ⅛ tsp cardamom, optional

DIRECTIONS:
1. Set the oven to 350°F.
2. In an oven-safe dish, combine the apricots with the coconut oil and cardamom (if using).
3. Bake the dish for 20 to 25 minutes, stirring once or twice, in a 350°F oven.

NUTRITION: Calories: 97; Carbs: 12.4 g; Protein: 0.5 g; Fat: 5.0 g

75. Chia Berry Smoothie

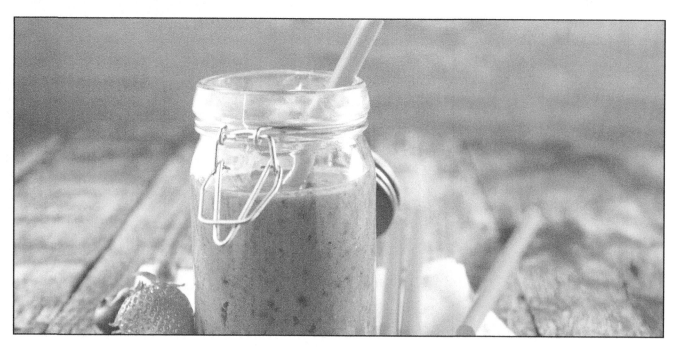

PREPARATION TIME: 10 minutes
COOKING TIME: 0 minutes
SERVINGS: 2
INGREDIENTS:

- 1 cup frozen pitted cherries, no-added-sugar
- ¼ cup fresh, or frozen, raspberries
- ¾ cup coconut water
- 1 Tbsp raw honey or maple syrup
- 1 tsp chia seeds
- 1 tsp hemp seeds
- Drop vanilla extract
- Ice

DIRECTIONS:

1. Combine in a blender the cherries, raspberries, coconut water, honey, chia seeds, hemp seeds, vanilla and ice. Blend until smooth.

NUTRITION: Calories: 139; Carbs: 25.2 g; Protein: 3.1 g; Fat: 3.2 g.

76. Green Detox Smoothie

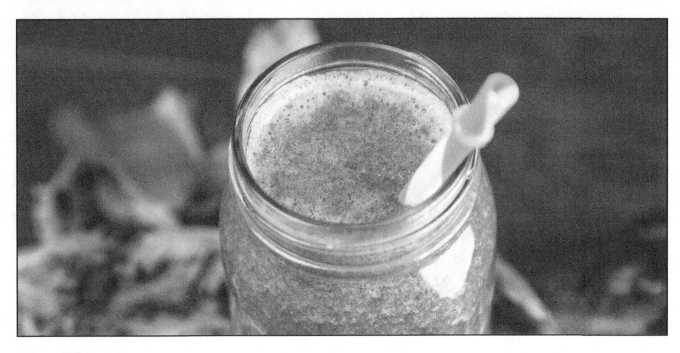

 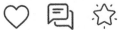

PREPARATION TIME: 5 minutes
COOKING TIME: 0 minutes
SERVINGS: 2
INGREDIENTS:
- ¾ to 1 cup water
- 1 cup spinach leaves
- 2 kale leaves
- 2 romaine lettuce leaves
- ½ avocado
- 1 pear

DIRECTIONS:
1. Combine the water, spinach, avocado, kale, romaine lettuce and pear in a blender. Serve after blending until smooth.

NUTRITION: Calories: 188; Carbs: 15.2 g; Protein: 3.7 g; Fat: 12.6 g.

77. Turmeric Smoothie

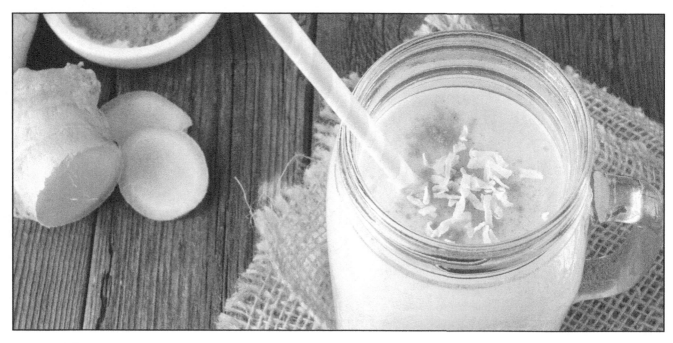

 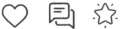   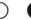

PREPARATION TIME: 5 minutes
COOKING TIME: 0 minutes
SERVINGS: 2
INGREDIENTS:

- 2 cups unsweetened almond milk
- 1 cup blueberries
- 2 Tbsp cocoa powder
- 1 to 2 packets Stevia
- 1 (1-inch) piece turmeric
- 1 cup crushed ice

DIRECTIONS:

1. Blend the almond milk, blueberries, cocoa powder, stevia, turmeric and ice in a blender. Blend until completely smooth.

NUTRITION: Calories: 78; Carbs: 9.4 g; Protein: 4.5 g; Fat: 2.6 g.

78. Carrot and Ginger Smoothie

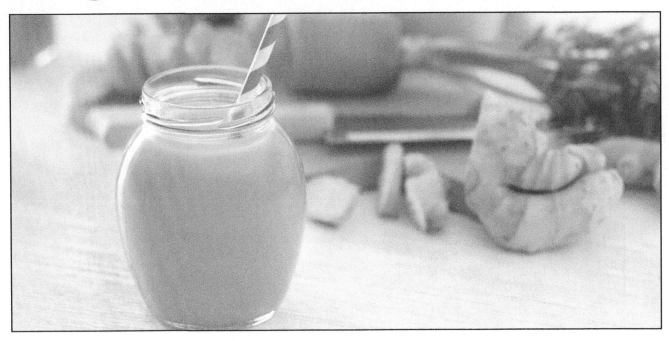

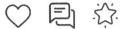

PREPARATION TIME: 10 minutes
COOKING TIME: 10 minutes
SERVINGS: 2
INGREDIENTS:
- ½ cup coconut milk
- ½ cup coconut water
- ¼ avocado
- ¼ cup unsweetened coconut shreds or flakes
- 1 tsp raw honey or maple syrup
- 1 thin slice fresh ginger
- 2 carrots
- Pinch ground cardamom (optional)
- Ice (optional)

DIRECTIONS:
1. Blend the coconut milk, coconut water, coconut, carrots, honey, avocado, ginger, cardamom (if used), and ice until smooth. Blend until completely smooth

NUTRITION: Calories: 246; Carbs: 16.2 g; Protein: 4.8 g; Fat: 18.1 g.

79. Avocado and Kale Smoothie

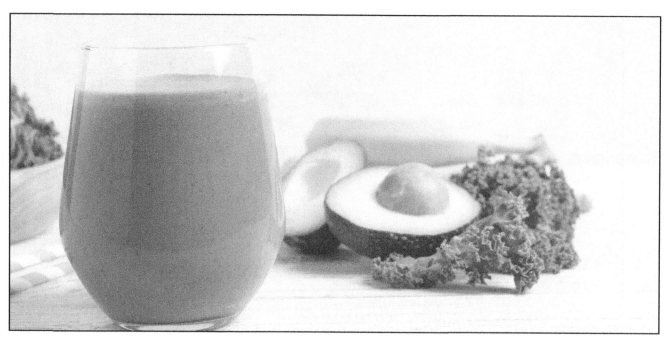

 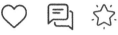 　　　　

PREPARATION TIME: 10 minutes
COOKING TIME: 0 minutes
SERVINGS: 2
INGREDIENTS:

- 2 cups fresh kale, tough ribs removed and chopped
- 2 celery stalks, chopped
- ½ avocado, peeled, pitted and chopped
- 1 (½-inch) piece fresh ginger root, chopped
- 1 (½-inch) piece fresh turmeric root, chopped
- 1 ½ cups unsweetened coconut milk
- ¼ cup ice cubes

DIRECTIONS:

1. In a high-power blender, add all the ingredients and pulse until smooth and creamy.
2. Transfer the smoothie into 2 serving glasses and serve immediately.

NUTRITION: Calories: 299; Carbs: 8.5 g; Protein: 4.4 g; Fat: 27.7 g.

80. Alkaline Papaya Smoothie

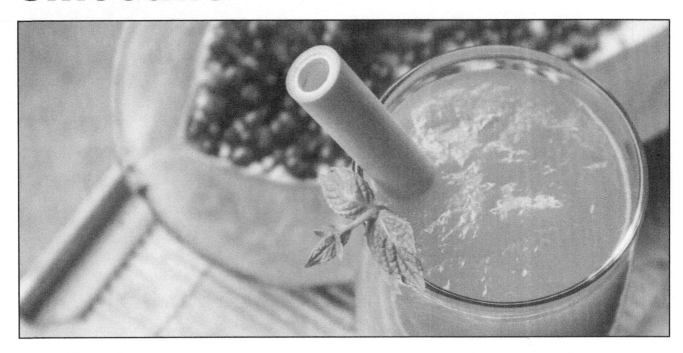

 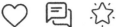   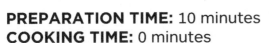

PREPARATION TIME: 10 minutes
COOKING TIME: 0 minutes
SERVINGS: 2
INGREDIENTS:

- ½ large papaya with seeds
- 4–5 dates
- 2 burro bananas
- ½ lb fresh spring water
- 1 Tbsp Bromide Plus Powder
- Juice ½ a key lime

DIRECTIONS:

1. Preheat the oven to 350°F (180°c).
2. Add all the ingredients to a bowl, mixing well.
3. Spread the nuts evenly on a rimmed baking sheet, baking until lightly toasted, about 10 to 15 minutes.
4. Set aside until cool completely.
5. Enjoy.

NUTRITION: Calories: 188; Carbs: 4.8 g; Protein: 6.1 g; Fat: 16.2 g.

81. Watermelon Smoothie

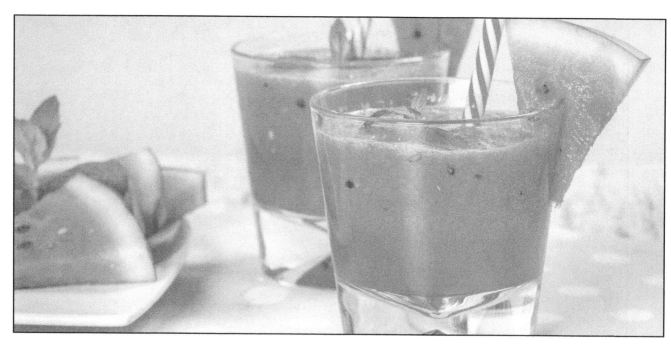

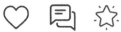   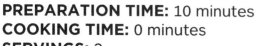

PREPARATION TIME: 10 minutes
COOKING TIME: 0 minutes
SERVINGS: 2
INGREDIENTS:
- 4 cups watermelon, seeded, cubed
- 4 key limes, juiced
- 4 cucumbers, seeded, sliced

DIRECTIONS:
1. Take a high-powered blender, switch it on, and then place all the ingredients inside, in order.
2. Cover the blender with its lid and then pulse at high speed for 1 minute or more.

NUTRITION: Calories: 71; Carbs: 16.1 g; Protein: 1.4 g; Fat: 0 g.

82. Mango and Pineapple Smoothie

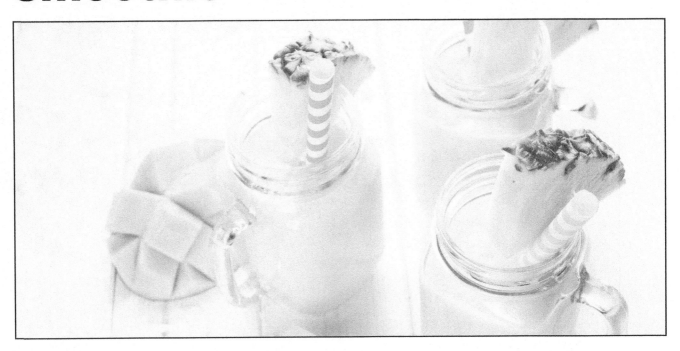

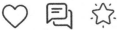

PREPARATION TIME: 10 minutes
COOKING TIME: 0 minutes
SERVINGS: 2
INGREDIENTS:

- 1 ¼ cup mango, peeled, pitted, and chopped
- 1 cup pineapple, peeled and chopped
- 1 Tbsp chia seeds
- 1 tsp ground turmeric
- ½ tsp ground ginger
- ½ tsp ground cinnamon
- Pinch vanilla powder
- 1 tsp coconut oil
- 1 cup unsweetened coconut milk
- ½ cup ice cubes

DIRECTIONS:

1. In a high-power blender, add all the ingredients and pulse until smooth and creamy.
2. Transfer the smoothie into 2 serving glasses and serve immediately.

NUTRITION: Calories: 337; Carbs: 28.1 g; Protein: 4.3 g; Fat: 23.0 g.

83. Yummy Cherry Smoothie

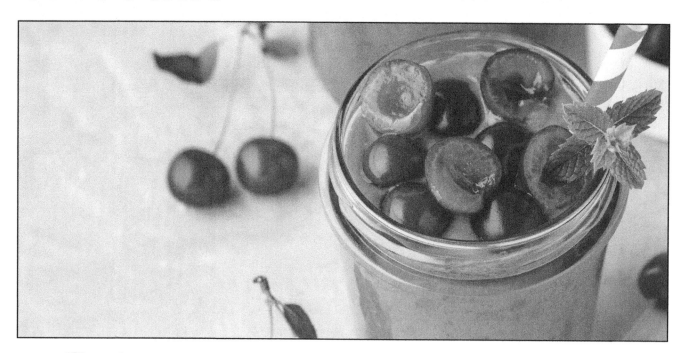

 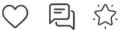

PREPARATION TIME: 10 minutes
COOKING TIME: 0 minutes
SERVINGS: 2
INGREDIENTS:
- 1 cup frozen no-added-sugar pitted cherries
- ¼ cup raspberries
- ¾ cup coconut water
- 1 Tbsp raw honey or maple syrup
- 1 tsp chia seeds
- 1 tsp hemp seeds
- Drop vanilla extract
- ice (optional)

DIRECTIONS:
1. Blend the cherries, raspberries, coconut water, honey, chia seeds, hemp seeds, vanilla and ice in a blender until smooth (if using). Blend until completely smooth.

NUTRITION: Calories: 163; Carbs: 27.4 g; Protein: 3.1 g; Fat: 4.5 g

Chapter 5:

12-Week Meal Plan

DAYS	BREAKFAST	LUNCH/DINNER	DESSERT/SNACK
WEEK 1			
1	Berry breakfast shake	Veggie and Hummus Sandwich	Pumpkin pie
	Zucchini, Corn and Egg Casserole	Black Bean Quinoa Bowl	
2	Spinach Smoothie	Lentil Salad	Blueberry muffins
3	Banana Oatmeal	Sandwiches with green salad, avocado, cucumber, and cheese	Carrot cake with dark chocolate
4	Whole grain French toast with pumpkin	Veggie burgers with beans and vegetables	Quinoa and chocolate cookies
5	Chia Breakfast	Veggie Lunch Salad	Lemon semi-integral flour plum cake
6	Greek yogurt with fresh berries and granola	Healthy Golden Eggplant Fries	Anti-inflammatory Lemon Bars
7	Peaches Baked With Cream Cheese	Saucy Garlic Greens	Chocolate Muffins

WEEK 2			
1	Baked Rice Porridge with Maple and Fruit	Delicious Vegetarian Lasagna	Poppy Seed Cake
2	Walnuts Granola For Breakfast	Chicken and quinoa salad with spinach and lettuce	Aromatic Cherry tart
3	Pumpkin Pancakes	Grilled salmon with white bean salad	Baked sweet potato chips
4	Blueberry Breakfast Blend	Vegetable Spring Roll Wraps	Dried banana chips
5	Fruit and Millet Breakfast	Curry Carrot Soup	Roasted chickpeas
6	Chia berry smoothie	Easy Broccoli Salad	Superfoods bars with a mix of nuts and seeds
7	Green detox smoothie	Lemony Feta and Lentil Salad	Peanut Butter Protein Bars

WEEK 3

1	Turmeric smoothie	Tabbouleh	Beet Chips	
2	Carrot and ginger smoothie	Chicken curry served in a pan	Garlic Oyster Crackers	
3		Carrot soup with whole-grain croutons	Butternut fries	
4	Avocado and Kale Smoothie	Grilled salmon steak	Date-ginger bars	
5	Alkaline Papaya Smoothie	Farro salad with cucumbers.	Zucchini chips	
6	Cherry Smoothie	Root Vegetable Loaf	Roasted apricots	
7	Watermelon Smoothie	French Soup	Pumpkin pie	

WEEK 4

1	Mango and Pineapple Smoothie	Thai Cauliflower Rice Salad with Peanut Butter Sauce		
2	Cherry Smoothie	Black Bean Soup	Blueberry muffins	
3	Berry breakfast shake	Parmesan-Crusted Scallops and Greens	Carrot cake with dark chocolate	
4	Zucchini, Corn and Egg Casserole	Alkaline Chili non Carne	Quinoa and chocolate cookies	
5	Spinach Smoothie	The Healthy Fish Tacos	Lemon semi integral flour plum cake	
6	Banana Oatmeal	Cod fillet with herbs	Anti-inflammatory Lemon Bars	
7	Whole grain French toast with pumpkin	Roasted cauliflower with cheese	Chocolate Muffins	

WEEK 5

1	Chia Breakfast	Mexican quinoa and lemon salad	Poppy Seed Cake
2	Greek yogurt with fresh berries and granola	Beet and bean burgers	Aromatic Cherry tart
3	Peaches Baked With Cream Cheese	Grilled mackerel with asparagus	Baked sweet potato chips
4	Baked Rice Porridge with Maple and Fruit	Tempeh With Olives And Capers	Dried banana chips
5	Walnuts Granola For Breakfast	Rolls Of Quinoa Lettuce And Raspberries	Roasted chickpeas
6	Pumpkin Pancakes	Oven Roasted Root Vegetables with Honey	Superfoods bars with mix of nuts and seeds
7	Blueberry Breakfast Blend	Red Lentils with Spinach Bars	Peanut Butter Protein Bars

WEEK 6

1	Fruit and Millet Breakfast	Broccoli and cheese casserole	Beet Chips
2	Chia berry smoothie	Baked potatoes stuffed with vegetables	Garlic Oyster Crackers
3	Green detox smoothie	Green curry	Butternut fries
4	Turmeric smoothie	Shrimp in curry sauce	Date-ginger bars
5	Carrot and ginger smoothie	Roasted Broccoli and Ham Casserole	Zucchini chips
6		Italian Eggplant Casserole	Roasted apricots
7	Avocado and Kale Smoothie	Butternut Squash Casserole	Pumpkin pie

WEEK 7

1	Alkaline Papaya Smoothie	Eggplant Parmesan Casserole	
2	Watermelon Smoothie	Veggie and Hummus Sandwich	Blueberry muffins
3	Mango and Pineapple Smoothie	Black Bean Quinoa Bowl	Carrot cake with dark chocolate
4	Cherry Smoothie	Lentil Salad	Quinoa and chocolate cookies
5	Berry breakfast shake	Sandwiches with green salad, avocado, cucumber and cheese	Lemon semi-integral flour plum cake
6	Zucchini, Corn and Egg Casserole	Veggie burgers with beans and vegetables	Anti-inflammatory Lemon Bars
7	Spinach Smoothie	Veggie Lunch Salad	Chocolate Muffins

WEEK 8

1	Banana Oatmeal	Healthy Golden Eggplant Fries	Poppy Seed Cake
2	Whole grain French toast with pumpkin	Saucy Garlic Greens	Aromatic Cherry tart
3	Chia Breakfast	Delicious Vegetarian Lasagna	Baked sweet potato chips
4	Greek yogurt with fresh berries and granola	Chicken and quinoa salad with spinach and lettuce	Dried banana chips
5	Peaches Baked With Cream Cheese	Grilled salmon with white bean salad	Roasted chickpeas
6	Baked Rice Porridge with Maple and Fruit	Vegetable Spring Roll Wraps	Superfoods bars with mix of nuts and seeds
7	Walnuts Granola For Breakfast	Curry Carrot Soup	Peanut Butter Protein Bars

WEEK 9

1	Pumpkin Pancakes	Easy Broccoli Salad	Beet Chips
2	Blueberry Breakfast Blend	Lemony Feta and Lentil Salad	Garlic Oyster Crackers
3	Fruit and Millet Breakfast	Tabbouleh	Butternut fries
4	Chia berry smoothie	Chicken curry served in a pan	Date-ginger bars
5	Green detox smoothie	Carrot soup with whole-grain croutons	Zucchini chips
6	Turmeric smoothie	Grilled salmon steak	Roasted apricots
7	Carrot and ginger smoothie	Farro salad with cucumbers.	Pumpkin pie

WEEK 10

1		Root Vegetable Loaf	
2	Avocado and Kale Smoothie	French Soup	Blueberry muffins
3	Alkaline Papaya Smoothie	Thai Cauliflower Rice Salad with Peanut Butter Sauce	Carrot cake with dark chocolate
4	Watermelon Smoothie	Black Bean Soup	Quinoa and chocolate cookies
5	Mango and Pineapple Smoothie	Parmesan-Crusted Scallops and Greens	Lemon semi-integral flour plum cake
6	Cherry Smoothie	Alkaline Chili non-Carne	Anti-inflammatory Lemon Bars
7	Berry breakfast shake	The Healthy Fish Tacos	Chocolate Muffins

WEEK 11 AND 12			
1	Zucchini, Corn and Egg Casserole	Cod fillet with herbs	Poppy Seed Cake
2	Spinach Smoothie	Roasted cauliflower with cheese	Aromatic Cherry tart
3	Banana Oatmeal	Mexican quinoa and lemon salad	Baked sweet potato chips
4	Whole grain French toast with pumpkin	Beet and bean burgers	Dried banana chips
5	Chia Breakfast	Grilled mackerel with asparagus	Roasted chickpeas
6	Greek yogurt with fresh berries and granola	Tempeh With Olives And Capers	Superfoods bars with a mix of nuts and seeds
7	Peaches Baked With Cream Cheese	Rolls Of Quinoa Lettuce And Raspberries	Peanut Butter Protein Bars

8	Baked Rice Porridge with Maple and Fruit	Oven Roasted Root Vegetables with Honey	Beet Chips
9	Walnuts Granola For Breakfast	Red Lentils with Spinach	Garlic Oyster Crackers
10	Pumpkin Pancakes	Broccoli and cheese casserole	Butternut fries
11	Blueberry Breakfast Blend	Baked potatoes stuffed with vegetables	Date-ginger bars
12	Fruit and Millet Breakfast	Green curry	Zucchini chips
13	Berry breakfast shake	Shrimp in curry sauce	Roasted apricots
14	Zucchini, Corn and Egg Casserole	Roasted Broccoli and Ham Casserole	Pumpkin pie

Chapter 11:

FAQ

HERE ARE JUST A FEW OF THE QUESTIONS AND ANSWERS THAT HAVE EMERGED THROUGH THE NUMEROUS INTERVIEWS CONDUCTED WITH OUR FANS AND READERS.

- I'm trying to figure out why I have such a strong reaction when I drink wine. This has only occurred since I stopped eating inflammatory foods (now for about 4 months.) The same thing happens when I eat a small sugary pastry or a slice of cake.Since I've been sugar-free, it's almost as if my body can't handle ANY sugar.Has anyone else had this happen to them? Have I over-purified my body to the point where I now have ZERO tolerance?

I will never drink wine again, despite the fact that I live 40 minutes from Napa Valley. My body will never tolerate it again; the reaction is so unpleasant that I don't want it. I'm also extremely sensitive to all types of sugar, including fruit. Because of this, I only use berries in my smoothies. Understanding your own body is essential for success with inflammation. It makes no difference what works for others; it is simply a tool for using suggestions to get to know your own self.

When you consume inflammatory foods on a regular basis, your body becomes accustomed to them and the pain response becomes less severe (but many health problems). When you eat clean and reintroduce inflammatory foods, your body reacts much more severely, and you can feel the inflammatory pain.

Fruit sugars are not as easily absorbed as processed sugars. Sugar is used by your body to produce free fatty acids. Free fatty acids are to blame for inflammation in the body. Processed sugar's chemical breakdown is ideal for inducing inflammation. The chemical breakdown of natural sugar tends to stick to other molecules, making it more difficult for your body to use to produce free fatty acids, implying that inflammation is more difficult to produce.

I never thought processed sugars would be better, but they do keep you hooked because they hit the brain faster, providing a feel-good dopamine hit. You may feel better while using it because it feeds the bad bacteria, but when you stop using it, these bacteria have nothing to feed on and you will feel worse for quite some time. However, the amount of fruit you consume is excessive. Perhaps it would be better to focus on more vegetables for the time being.

Fiber does not accompany bad sugars. Fruit contains fiber, which allows the body to process it more quickly and differently. Bad sugars cause an increase in sugar consumption, which leads to high blood sugar and a pro-inflammatory state.

A high-sugar diet may feed inflammatory bacteria in the gut preferentially. Sugar (especially fructose) can cause the liver to produce toxic levels of fat Because it is processed more slowly and differently. — I work as a nutritional health coach.

The Fodmap diet explains how different sugars break down in your body and what to avoid until you figure out your tolerance.

One of my first GERD symptoms was my aversion to red wine. I had no idea what fresh new hell that would wreak at the time. I'm no longer able to consume wine.

I too, am unable to handle alcohol. I can have one gentle glass and be fine, but it's always a risk and not worth it on a regular basis. Although my joints prompted me to adopt an AI lifestyle, alcohol does not even pass through my body to cause inflammation in them. My body simply rejects the alcohol, and I vomit for hours... hurray! My friend gets a sugar hangover after eating too much melon. Ah, the joys of being in tune.

I can only drink red wines with the lowest histamine levels, such as Beaujolais, Pinot, or Gamay noir. Otherwise, my rosacea, GERD, nausea, and migraines will be ready to go!

- My family is already on a tight budget, and it appears that substitutes are prohibitively expensive. Can anyone assist me in creating a list that won't break the bank?

Rather than looking for processed/packaged substitutes, I've discovered that using simple, whole ingredients whenever possible is often less expensive. Vegetables, fruits, and lentils/legumes (if they do not irritate you). Then splurge on just 1–2 substitute items, such as pasta and bread.

Consume real food. Certain fruits and vegetables are on sale every week at most supermarkets, or frozen is also good and usually not expensive... Just don't eat anything that has been frozen. Beans are inexpensive, especially if you buy a bag of dried beans and cook them yourself.

Everyone here is correct. Maintain simplicity. Each of our meals includes some meat and steamed vegetables. As well as fruits for snacking. On occasion, gluten-free pasta is used. The following are the results of a survey. My husband smokes everything and we freeze it in family-size portions. Following that, grocery trips consist of fruits and vegetables. I never spend more than $50 per week on groceries for our family. This method has made mealtimes so much easier for me. And I've discovered that the entire family has adapted to "eat to live" rather than "live to eat." You can't go wrong with fresh vegetables, grass-fed ground beef, chicken, ground turkey, dried beans, peas, bone broth, instant pot GF pasta that isn't too pricey, and brown rice and quinoa can be meal stretchers.

I don't do any kind of substitutions. If you're looking for low-cost meals, dried beans, chicken, and soup are all options.

Purchasing simple, unprocessed foods is far less expensive than purchasing ready-made and packaged foods. We eat whole grains, seeds, a little low-fat dairy, olive oil and ghee, vegetables, fruit, legumes, and very little animal protein (chicken, turkey, fish). Dealing with multiple issues and this plan appear to be the most effective.

Frozen vegetables! Much less expensive and will not spoil.

I understand. Purchasing real food is prohibitively expensive. Because they can only afford cheap pasta and other foods, most poor people are overweight. When chicken or turkey is on sale, I try to buy large packs and freeze them. Broccoli and green beans are usually inexpensive, and frozen vegetables are frequently on sale. Chickpeas are typically inexpensive and can be used to make hummus. Eggs are not too expensive, and I buy large containers of Greek yogurt, nuts, and brown rice in bulk. Apples and bananas are reasonably priced. Tuna and chicken in can go on sale.

Cook in a pan with a blob of real natural butter, seasonings, a can of puréed tomato, and some diced onion... My boys enjoy it with a fried egg or scrambled egg and fresh, crunchy shredded lettuce. I like it with sautéed shredded green cabbage.

I use mayonnaise in place of sour cream in any dish that calls for creaminess. It's certainly less expensive than sour cream substitutes. Plus, making your own is simple and inexpensive. Then you'll know what ingredients are in it. Cassava flour is inexpensive and works well as a substitute for wheat flour if you can tolerate it. Of course, it is slightly more expensive than wheat flour, but it goes a long way.

Kids can help chop and prepare whole fresh vegetables, which are healthier and less expensive.

When I have time, I make my own GF crackers as well as homemade granola-better for you made with pure maple syrup, no sugar and dried fruits and nuts.

- Is it wheat that causes inflammation, or is it gluten in wheat that causes inflammation?

Will switching to gluten-free foods, such as gluten-free bread and pasta, help? I'm attempting to alter my diet in order to alleviate joint pain. I'm also avoiding milk in favor of soya or almond milk, and I'm attempting to avoid sugar as well. Starting to-morrow.

Gluten is a major cause of my joint pain, and I've discovered that "gluten-free" products aren't much better due to all the added ingredients like bad oils and sugar. There are many different kinds of people. I mostly eat vegetables, fruit, healthy fats, and high-quality protein from Whole Foods. I also discovered that it wasn't just about food; I needed to manage stress, sleep better, and improve my detox pathways.

Eliminating gluten, dairy, and nightshades (tomato, eggplant, white potato, and capsicum) aided my recovery.

I don't have an issue with gluten or dairy, but rather with refined, fried, and oily foods.

The majority of people are not gluten sensitive. Most people can tolerate whole wheat. Sprouted is preferable. Trader Joe's has several sprouted whole grain bread that have little or no sugar. My favorite is their Daily Bread. If you are sensitive to gluten, they also have gluten-free whole-grain bread.

It all depends on the individual. I can also work with Einkorn flour, which is more flavorful (low gluten, organic primitive wheat made in Italy can only find on Amazon though). Most people who are gluten intolerant can. Find a good bakery or make your own gluten-free bread. The term "candy store" refers to a store that sells candy. Oat milk is my favorite. Many people are allergic to soy. I'm not bothered by almonds.

Different people react differently to wheat, gluten, and even yeast. But going gluten-free is a good place to start; it changed my life in a matter of days. As previously stated, many gluten-free foods contain additives, so look for alternatives such as quinoa, buckwheat, and wild rice. Learn to read ingredient lists; a good rule of thumb is that if you've never heard of an ingredient, you probably don't want to eat it. Consider eating more from scratch and avoiding processed/packaged foods. When I first started eating anti-inflammatory foods, I made a simple list of foods that I tested to see if they were inflammatory.

It's gluten, and it's found in foods other than wheat. BROW stands for barley, rye, oats, and wheat (all forms). Use almond milk instead of soy milk, which is highly inflammatory.

- I'm literally crying because I've been losing weight quickly since starting this diet. The problem is that I used to love my body (at least some of it), but now I feel really unattractive. How can I put on weight?

I'm avoiding wheat, dairy, and tomatoes, and I was SUPPOSED to avoid potatoes, but I decided to eat them in order to regain my weight. I make a smoothie or porridge daily with almond milk, peanut butter, and flax seed. What other types of smoothies are available? I'm also trying to eat an avocado several times per week. Portion sizes are small ISH right now because I've completely lost my appetite and am working hard to regain it.

Adding hemp seeds, chia seeds, and/or peanut

butter to smoothies increases protein and calories, as do healthy fats like avocado, coconut oil, and fish oil. Protein powders can be beneficial, but keep an eye out for the sugar content.

Protein shakes are similar to weight gainers. Whey protein isolate is lactose-free and anti-inflammatory for many people. You can have one after a meal or before bedtime before you feel full. You can buy them unsweetened and unflavored and flavor them yourself. Depending on your tolerance, you can also begin to increase your consumption of extra-virgin olive oil, butter, and nuts. Too much fat at first may upset your digestive system, but gradually increasing your fat intake will allow your body to adapt. These are high-calorie foods in small quantities.

Look up a chocolate avocado smoothie recipe. I used to make one with bananas, avocados, cocoa powder, peanut butter, and a few other ingredients. It was delicious but extremely fatty and high in calories.

Nuts, nut butter, healthy oils, muffins, pancakes, sweet potatoes, pea protein in smoothies, hemp hearts, pumpkin seeds, flax seeds, and coconut milk are all high in calories.

I lost weight after covid and haven't had my appetite since June! So I started taking probiotics, and it's all better now.

- My doctor says I'm pre-diabetic and have a lot of inflammation. I stopped drinking soda, which was easier than I expected. I'm just having difficulty figuring out meal planning. I've never been a big meat eater, so I struggle to get enough protein. I like salmon and tilapia, but I'm not sure if I can eat them every day. I'm okay with eggs, depending on how they're cooked.

Unfortunately, there is no single answer; it is trial and error until you find a method that works for you. Some people here have acute inflammation caused by specific foods, whereas others, like me, have low-grade whole-body chronic inflammation that may or may not 'flare' after eating certain foods, but eliminating the most common inflammatory foods helps. The most important 'rule' for me is to avoid processed foods. Anything from a box or packet, all dairy (except Greek yogurt, which I eat for probiotic purposes), all commercially farmed meat (fed on wheat and full of artificial hormones, etc.), and no refined foods such as white bread, pasta, noodles, or white rice. Consume wholegrain foods with low GI and plenty of fruits and vegetables. Yes, please, to fish and seafood.

A meal should consist of one meat (chicken, fish, eggs, etc.) and two vegetables. Once a day, berries or a small amount of fruit. Because of the metals they contain, fish should not be consumed on a daily basis. Once or twice a week is sufficient. For a quick meal, boil some eggs and mix in some vegetables and berries. Look into some low-carb meals as well.

Salmon is delicious, and I could eat it every day. Breakfast is difficult for me, but thinking outside the box allows that salmon to satisfy my morning hunger as well. According to what I've learned, eggs are highly inflammatory for me.

For breakfast, I used to make a salad with oven-baked chicken breast (pre-prepared), green leaves, an avocado, and some cherry tomatoes, drizzled with olive oil and lime juice. It keeps me satisfied for at least 5 hours.

I went to the library and borrowed anti-inflammatory cookbooks. To get a sense of what is possible. Eliminating sugar (including alcohol), dairy, red meat, beans, and all grains except quinoa is a good place to start to give your stomach a rest. If you haven't had a gut test, this will help you pinpoint where you might be having a problem so you can focus your healing efforts. Starting with a daily probiotic and prebiotic can be beneficial.

Look up the glycemic index to see which carbs are less likely to cause a spike in your glucose levels. White rice, white potatoes, and cold cereals all spike quickly. It matters what carbs you eat and when you eat them.

Hello, you can also get protein from vegetables, such as lentils, chickpeas, and black/red beans. The highest protein content among meats is found in chicken breast, oats with berries and chopped walnuts, unsweetened coconut, and oat milk.

- I recently began to make the connection between sugar and severe joint pain. I have tendinitis in my feet, but my thumb is extremely swollen. I'm going to give it a shot and see how it goes.

Sugar is both horrible and addictive. I stopped (mostly) using it over 18 months ago, and my joint pain has subsided. I had a very sugary apple fritter yesterday, and I'm currently laying in front of my red light getting help for my knees. Sugar is the color of death. Natural sugars don't seem to bother me, though this could be because I don't o.d. on them. My body tolerates the addition of fruit and vegetables as well as fiber and healthy fat, to my smoothies.

Sugar is "concrete for the joints and digestive system," and I definitely associate sugar consumption with body pain. The only solution I've found is a clean diet rich in lean protein, vegetables, and fruits. Natural sugars in fruit do not bother me, but any refined sugar is a trigger. You will most likely spend the next six months learning how to read labels and discovering which foods you enjoy. Almost anything can be replaced with a good substitute. Dates, for example, are now like chocolate to me, and they use dates to sweeten a variety of foods.

The key is to read labels; you are correct about sugars. Making your own food is important and beneficial in every way.

- Do you have any suggestions for quitting sugar? I'm totally addicted to iced coffee!!

The only option for me is to quit cold turkey. It becomes easier after a few weeks, and fruits and vegetables begin to taste sweeter than before. For cravings, I reach for dates, figs, and super-ripe mangos... and try to avoid sweeteners, which only serve to keep you hooked on the sweet stuff.

It hurts at first, but it gets easier, and you'll be surprised at how much sweetness you can consume!

I've had success with natural sweeteners like honey and (real) maple syrup in small amounts. Lattes with honey-cinnamon-oat milk are delicious. I've never tried to ice one, but I'm sure it would be delicious!

Find something else that you enjoy. It also helps to keep yourself busy so you don't think about it.

I weened away because I was borderline diabetic, so I gradually reduced to fewer pumps of chocolate in my iced coffee, then to sugar-free, and when I had to go cold turkey, that's when I'd eat sugar and I'd immediately be in a lot of pain! My hands began to hurt, and my ankles began to hurt; not fun! I now make my own iced coffee and add coconut milk to it. I find alternative ways to treat myself without using refined sugar. Make use of raw, local honey, pure maple syrup, and date syrup. Truvani makes a good plant-based protein powder in vanilla or chocolate that is AI and adds a natural sweetness to things. There are so many good recipes on Pinterest that you can choose alternative ways to adapt without sugar. It's been a year on AI for me, and I still want to grab a bite of a donut or cake at work, but I try to resist and eat fruit instead!

I used to be a chocoholic, but thanks to the vitamins I take, I no longer crave. I'm taking a Costco multivitamin, 2 turmeric capsules, 1 vitamin D capsule, 2 calcium capsules, and 2 salmon oil capsules. My nails have also become hard.

- Have you tried Turmeric capsules for inflammation?

Black pepper, turmeric, and ginger. Combine in equal parts. Take on the tongue and swallow, or place in a shot glass of juice or water and drink. Beautiful

Yes, and I take 1500 mg twice a day; I notice a significant improvement in joint pain.

I've read that you can have too much. I'd recommend only every other day because I've read that you can get too much. I'd recommend using curcumin only every other day; it's been a lifesaver for my pain. I started taking it months before my prescription and my CRP levels dropped significantly to just above normal. Taking both a prescription and an herbal anti-inflammatory is definitely beneficial to me. I'm glad I have it now after having to discontinue my Rx due to serious side effects. I'm stiff and in pain, but nothing compared to when I had to stop everything for surgery in November.

Yes, I have, and they are excellent. The only disadvantage is that it thins the blood. If you have to have surgery, your blood becomes thin. It happened to me once, and the doctor asked if I was taking blood thinners because my blood had thinned and it was difficult to control the bleeding.

Yes. I was surprised that it helped me almost immediately, within two or three days. I had been suffering so much and I was perfectly normal. I bought a grocery store brand that was cheap and cheerful. Turmeric and black pepper. The irony is that I come from a culture that believes in drinking turmeric milk for pain and applying turmeric to wounds, among other things... I did that for a month or so, and I also fed the lattes to my elderly parents. That didn't seem to make a difference. I've only recently discovered this golden paste recipe and have yet to try it. Unfortunately, I have gallstones and am hesitant to take it. Edit: Initially, I was a regular because I was astounded by the outcome. That lasted about two months. I only take it now when I remember or when I feel that strange fatigue and pain.

I put ground turmeric in my tea, and it does help with pain, allergies, stuffiness, and headaches. For absorption, add black pepper. There are a lot of them.

- Are there any chips that are safe to eat on an anti-inflammatory diet, or should you avoid them all?

Consider Siete brand chips. They make tortilla chips and various potato chips. They are fried in avocado oil, so there are no seed wells, and the ingredients are very clean... And they taste great.

Homemade olive oil and salt chips

I'm not sure if it's appropriate for everyone, but I enjoy Avocado oil chips.

I discovered Jackson's sweet crisps with coconut oil or avocado. The same goes for plantain chips. There are also some cassava chips. It has a nice crunch to it with the salt.

- What are some AI foods that people eat that actually taste good?

Natural peanut butter with honey and apple slices

Almonds and pecans in their natural state. Larabars, apples with almond butter Just read the ingredients per flavor.

I enjoy pumpkin seeds. On a daily basis, I snack. Magnesium, fiber, and protein in abundance

On rice crackers, spread hummus with olives. Apple with a dollop of peanut butter on top. Toast with avocado. Fruit topped with almond milk whip.

I like my fresh vegetables plain, with hummus, or with guacamole. Every now and then, I allow myself a serving of animal crackers. I also enjoy cut-up apples and peaches.

Plantain and cassava chips served with hummus or guacamole. Smoothies, pistachios, and so on.

We snack on kale chips, apple chips, vegan queso, dates with peanut butter, dried figs, homemade trail mix, fruit, guacamole, pico de gallo, banana ice cream sandwiches, and wild blueberry oat bars, to name a few.

Look into Siete brand chips. Despite the fact that their potato chips are made from white potatoes, they are cooked in avocado oil, which is delicious. They have a dairy-free nacho cheese flavor that is absolutely delicious there. Tortilla chips are also delicious.

I'm a sucker for nuts and berries. My grown daughter shared that she warms frozen fruit (choose your favorite mix) and then adds chia seeds. I'll also toss in some pumpkin seeds or cashews. Allow them to sit for a few minutes to allow the chia to absorb the fruit juice before serving. I also snack on dried fruit and nuts to avoid added sugars. Apples with nut butter; I avoid peanut butter, but most other nut butters appear to be fine. Sliced avocado with tomatoes and pecans or almonds.

My first kompot was made with dried apricots and prunes. I threw in some apples. It was delectable. I even mixed it into my oatmeal.

Cucumbers, kefir cheese, mint, and olive oil

- Do eggs cause inflammation? I've heard that whites are

Hi. Eggs are inflammatory triggers because they can feed bacteria, viruses, and fungi. So, if the body is in the process of healing, it is best to avoid them for a while. The word on the street is that there is no such thing as a bad egg. It also depends on the egg. Is it a chicken or a duck egg? Although duck egg is very beneficial for liver support, it is not recommended for people who have digestive issues.

Yes, I eat organic because it appears to be healthier.

I switched to pasture-raised organic eggs and no longer had problems with them, but everyone is different.

The bottom line is that eggs are a superfood, so I'll keep eating organic-free range.

Eating eggs is a great way to get a good dose of protein into your diet. Contrary to popular belief, the American Heart Association now recognizes eggs as one of the healthiest foods you can eat, despite their bad reputation in the past. After eating eggs, you are unlikely to feel hungry for an extended period of time. Eggs contain all nine essential amino acids, making them a complete protein source. Eggs' high protein content makes them an excellent addition to any breakfast casserole recipe.

- For those of you who began an anti-inflammatory diet to help manage autoimmune disease pain, how long before you began to notice an improvement in pain and symptoms?

Hello, Debbie. It would be great to start to detox your body for a few days (3–7 days — no more during the winter time as your body needs more energy) (3–7 days — no more during the winter time as your body needs more energy). This absolutely gets rest to your homeostasis — and elimination organs can get completely reset. Your liver would get a better chance to remove accumulated toxins, heavy metals, or unwanted things. Also, fasting is not suitable for each body's constitution, so it would be better to avoid it unless you know exactly what is more beneficial than harmful. After then, you can start implementing your anti-inflammatory diet. Your body will be able to act quickly as you give a break to your digestive tract during the detox. You still have to eat but very plain diet — manageable for a few days but your results will be quicker. Inflammation is very individual because it depends on how much our main elimination channels (Liver, Kidney) are blocked.

Changing the water pH of foods you eat and letting go of stress can happen in days. The x39 stem cell patch is amazing to relieve pain and ache.

I started anti-inflammatory keto and 16/8 IF. I use the Bobby-approved app to make sure my ingredients are clean and anti-inflammatory. Almost immediately, I had improvements. The fasting has been a Godsend. My weight dropped 45 lbs in 2 months. I also supplement my gut cause most likely you have a leaky gut and that will affect every aspect of your body. I supplement my liver, thyroid, and adrenals. Once all my inflammation was gone, I found the main issue that I'm now working on. It was a fixed one that uncovered another situation for me. I think I found my root cause after everything. My goiter has shrunk, the nodules are gone, my COMPLETE labs are almost normal by functional standards and my adrenal fatigue is improving now that I found and am working on IBD.

Depends on the specific trigger. Certain substances can take a long time to detox from. Gluten it's something like 6 months. You can try adding supplements to help speed things along like DPP-IV.

Five to seven days. Depends on the severity and your pain tolerance. A rash I had for over 5 years is now completely gone and that took three weeks. Clearer skin for 4 weeks. Now when I try to put something back into my new way of living, I know within hours if it's going to have a bad reaction.

I stopped gluten first and felt better in a week. It's hard at first, but once you get your mind wrapped around it, it is easy.

I am not sure if I had withdrawals due to the diet change or if it was because I was also trying to quit smoking. I am on an alkaline vegan diet and I do know that my enzymes and bloodwork have improved in just 3 weeks of being on this diet.

- What do you all know about food sensitivity tests? I know there are different kinds and they each work a little differently.

I did 2 different ones and got all different answers except for gluten. So I'm not super confident in them. Dairy didn't show up either, but I feel that dairy bothers me

Do a food journal and write your reactions if you get any to start pinpointing the foods vs wrong ones.

They r very unreliable — I personally wouldn't waste my money. Better to do an actual food elimination diet like AIP to truly determine the foods best for your body.

- I was visiting family out of town, and I've eaten a lot of foods that inflamed me. Are there things I can do to flush those toxins out of my body more quickly? My joints haven't hurt for

months, but now I can feel that my knees are threatening to flare up on me. I'm worried.

Drink a ton of water. If you can take an Epsom salt bath, do that. Drink more water. May need another bath tomorrow. Ibuprofen may ease up the pain a bit.

Lots of water and sweat it out! Do something that makes you sweat. I used to use an electric blanket and several blankets to make myself sweat until I couldn't stand it anymore. Knocked me out of a flare every time.

Don't eat red meat, the liver is the organ that detoxifies the body, so it doesn't need help, but if you go back to your normal diet or try veggies, fruits, chicken and fish, the inflammation maybe go faster

- Confused about nuts — so walnuts, almonds, etc., are good I think? What about cashews? But no on peanuts — correct? Why? Just figuring it out!

Almonds have a skin that contains lectins. They are best for you if you soak them. They are also high in omega-6 fatty acids, which are critical for health but inflammatory if you consume too many. A lot of things have omega 6 in them, including eggs. I was making the mistake of using a lot of almonds and eggs as healthy fat sources. But I was eating too many and it was making me ache. I take it easy on almonds and eggs. I eat lots of egg whites, though!

It's the skin of the almonds that has the lectins. I just think if you're going to use almonds, just don't use them for everything. Like, don't drink almond milk, and then have almonds in your granola, and also make almond bread. Have some almonds that day, just not a lot. And make sure to watch your omega-6 intake that day as well. This is only on my radar because I was supplementing with the omega-3, omega-6, and omega-9 supplements, and I ached so badly. Until I learned about omega-6 and stopped it. Now I watch my food carefully.

Peanuts are a legume. They grow underground and so are understood to be higher in contaminants that cause inflammation. The others are tree nuts that don't get sprayed as much but also have a harder shell as a protective barrier. There may be other reasons as well, but growing conditions are a factor.

Funny, there isn't much negative I can find about peanuts... they are a top 5 nut, almonds and pistachios and Brazil nuts seem to get the most accolades... but all are healthy and delicious choices in moderation, it seems!

I'm not sure, I think everyone is different about what they can eat. I eat peanut butter as it's nut butter. I think nuts are ok to eat for most.

Peanuts aren't really a nut, and I think you may want to avoid them because of the high omega-6 content. Also, beware that any nut can be roasted with less-healthy vegetable oils, so definitely look at the ingredient labels!

Almonds and walnuts are very good for your brain health. Cashews should be in moderation.

If you do get Peanut Butter, be sure it's organic and has no other ingredients. I don't like peanut butter, but my husband loves it.

- I'll be going back to work next week, after an extended break between jobs, and I need some ideas for packed lunches. What are some of your favorite bring-to-work lunches?

Today I had a fruit and almond milk smoothie, a piece of almond flour pear cake, brown rice with chicken and coconut curry, almond flour crackers, and about a tsp of goat cheese (I'm trying to figure out if I can eat goat cheese. So far, the results are promising.)

Grilled chicken and rice with coconut aminos (none of these are inflammatory for me), which I make on the weekend or a soup or stew that can be eaten many days of the week.

I pack a cucumber and tomato salad almost daily with olive oil and dried oregano.

I always take a small container of fruit and a small container of veggies along with leftovers from the night before, a hardboiled egg or tuna salad

Chicken with Dill, boiled eggs, black olives...cucumbers with salt and pepper, corn chips with homemade bean dip (with chopped lettuce, tomato, and green peppers on top), Green peppers stuffed with rice, hamburger, seasoned spaghetti sauce. Just a few favorites.

I can tell you exactly what I have today. I always bring a Chomp beef jerky from Trader Joe's as a snack. Lunch is sweet potato and some squash and zucchini and some salmon. I do chicken too. I bring some plantain chips to have if I get hungry again or an apple to sit on my desk. Good luck! Keep meals simple and meal prep on Sundays, you'll be glad you did.

Usually, dinner leftovers with some fruit with pretzels and hummus dip or some type of pita chip

– What do you drink when you're tired of plain Water?

I like Dragon Fruit flavored Vitamin Water. I add about a 1/3 cup to my 20 oz glass. Flavors the water. I drink spring water.

I add a packet or two of True Lemon or True Lime to my water when it gets boring. I also drink organic green iced tea.

I boil water with fennel seeds, cumin seeds, ginger, and cinnamon stick. Drink it like warm tea with lemon or room temp. Amazing health benefits and awesome flavor. Another thing I throw slices of lemon or oranges with peel in my bottle... it helps with flavor and is refreshing all day long. Add fresh mint leaves...

Unsweetened decaf tea (HteaO has blueberry decaf if you live near a location) and decaf coffee. I also put lemon or pineapple in my water at times.

Green tea. I'm reading a book right now that says any carbonation, even in drinks like Bubly, is not good as the carbonic acid used to carbonate liquids has an unwelcome consequence for our digestion.

Black cherry or cherry limeade. 0 sugar, 0 calories, 0 caffeine. Super tasty and under $4 a case at Walmart. They don't cause me any pain when I drink them but add flavor to my drink options.

Homebrewed unsweetened iced tea — a combination of regular black tea and green tea or black tea and ginger tea

Earl Grey crème or fennel in a diffuser tea ball in ice water. It just lightly flavors it.

Sparkling water with a splash of pomegranate juice. Hot water with lemon. Cucumber water.

Teas like turmeric Chai and ginger, I start the morning with warm water, lemon, and a couple of shakes of Redmond's Real salt.

Coffee, water with ice and straw help me drink more, and adding cucumbers and lemon to it will also help! Pom Margaritas too, are my top 3 drinks I consume.

Water with lemon and honey. Coconut water with pineapple and lime. Tea, mushroom coffee. Cucumber and green apple water with mint. Ginger, honey, and ACV water.

- Can high inflammation be healed?

Yes! Our bodies are amazing once you know why they are getting inflammation

Not sure about total elimination. I think it's relative to how you feel.

Yes, but take a very long time

Conclusion

Thank you for making it to the end of this anti-inflammatory diet cookbook. Unhealthy lifestyle choices can lead to a variety of undesirable physical and mental issues. Most people are unaware of how much stress is placed on your mind and body when you do not have adequate levels of hormones and vitamins that come with living a healthy lifestyle.

Chronic inflammation is increasingly being identified as the primary cause of civilization's diseases, including most cancers, heart disease, diabetes, obesity, and many others.

An anti-inflammatory diet is a way of life that consists of selecting and preparing foods that reduce inflammation based on scientific knowledge of how they can help your body achieve optimal health. Pay close attention to those that require you to eliminate an entire food group; many diets do this to ensure that you lose weight quickly, but as we've discussed in the book, it's better to lose weight slowly and in a healthy way than to lose weight quickly and unhealthily. Allowing others to influence your life requires caution.

Create solutions that are as realistic as possible. Remember that any positive change is sufficient. You are not required to make drastic changes all at once. Starting small can be the most beneficial way to get started in some cases. Remember that it is never too late to start, and if something isn't working for your health, try something else. Life is far too short to be spent in agony.

You will not only improve your personal well-being if you take the initiative and make the necessary health changes, such as proper diet choices, regular exercise, and a positive thought process, but you will also improve the lives of those around you.

Making a change can be challenging at times, but remember that your decisions affect more than just yourself; by incorporating this diet into your life, you are contributing to a healthier and more vibrant world. May this book bless you by inspiring new healthy ideas and guiding you on the path to perfect health.

Making healthy dietary choices and engaging in regular physical activity can provide greater benefits compared to relying solely on medication to address health issues.

Take things slowly and patiently. Your inflammation will not go away overnight. Simply start and watch the results for yourself. The first step is to identify your objectives. You've taken the first step toward a healthier lifestyle when you reach your goal.

An anti-inflammatory diet is effective because it includes a variety of foods rich in anti-inflammatory nutrients such as omega-3 fatty acids and antioxidants. Furthermore, avoid processed foods, alcohol, salt, sugar, trans fats, saturated fats, and tobacco products, as they can all worsen inflammation without providing any benefits.

If you are considering an anti-inflammatory diet, you should think twice about taking anti-inflammatory medications. Despite the AHA's lack of official endorsement, it's a good idea to be aware of this and avoid or limit your exposure to products that contain general inflammation if you have heart disease. NSAIDs (such as aspirin or acetaminophen), over-the-counter pain relievers such as ibuprofen, and other antihypertensive medications are just a few examples of what can cause inflammation.

Good luck with your new diet.

Bibliography

https://www.who.int/chp/chronic_disease_report/full_report.pdf

https://www.ncbi.nlm.nih.gov/pubmed?Db=pubmedandCmd=ShowDetailViewandTermToSearch=21195808

https://www.ncbi.nlm.nih.gov/pubmed?Db=pubmedandCmd=ShowDetailViewandTermToSearch=21195808

https://www.cancer.gov/about-cancer/causes-prevention/risk/chronic-inflammation

https://www.ncbi.nlm.nih.gov/pmc/articles/PMC5507106/

Marshall, cup (n.d.). Run Out of Curry Leaves? Here are the Best Substitutes – The Kitchen Community. The Kitchen Community. Retrieved February 25, 2022, from https:

//thekitchencommunity.org/substitutes-for-curry-leaves/

Martin, A. (2019, September). The Top 14 Healthiest Greens for Your Salad | Everyday Health. Everydayhealth.com. Https: //www.everydayhealth.com/diet-nutrition- pictures/best-salad-greens-for-your-health.aspx

Masters, R. cup, Liese, A. D., Haffner, S. M., Wagenknecht, L. E., and Hanley, A. J. (2010). Whole and Refined Grain Intakes Are Related to Inflammatory Protein: Concentrations in Human Plasma. The Journal of Nutrition: 140(3), 587–594. Https:

//doi.org/10.3945/jn.109.116640

Mayo Clinic Staff. (2020, October 14). Water: How much should you drink every day? Mayo Clinicup https: //www.mayoclinicuporg/healthy-lifestyle/nutrition-and-healthy- eating/in-depth/water/art-20044256

McDonald MD, E. (2020, September). What foods cause or reduce inflammation?

Www.uchicagomedicine.org.Https:

//www.uchicagomedicine.org/forefront/gastrointestinal-articles/what-foods-cause-or- reduce-inflammation

Medlineplus.(2017).Aminoacids:medlineplusMedicalEncyclopedia. Medlineplus.gov. Https: //medlineplus.gov/ency/article/002222.htm

Melanie. (2016, June 28). Delicious Salad Recipe to Reduce Inflammation. Remedy Physical Therapy. Https: //remedypt.com/8-delicious-salad-recipes-to-reduce- inflammation/

Meyer, H. (2018, June). Berry-Banana Cauliflower Smoothie. Eatingwell. Https:

//www.eatingwell.com/recipe/265882/berry-banana-cauliflower-smoothie/

Natto, Z. S., Yaghmoor, W., Alshaeri, H. K., and Van Dyke, T. E. (2019). Omega-3 Fatty Acids Effects on Inflammatory Biomarkers and Lipid Profiles among Diabetic and Cardiovascular Disease Patients: A Systematic Review and Meta-Analysis. Scientific Reports, 9(1). Https: //doi.org/10.1038/s41598-019-54535-x

Nevins, S. (2016, June 6). Tomato Basil Garlic Chicken. A Saucy Kitchen. Https:

//go.redirectingat.com/?Id=74679X1524629andsref=https%3A%2F%2Fwww.buzzfeed.com%2Fmichelleno%2F18-anti-inflammatory-recipes-that-will-make-you-feel betterandurl=https%3A%2F%2Fwww.asaucykitchen.com%2Ftomato-basil-garlic- chicken%2Fandxcust=5020798%7C%7CAMP%7C0andxs=1

Nutrition: cup for F. S. And A. (2022). Advice about Eating Fish. FDA. Https:

//www.fda.gov/food/consumers/advice-about-eating-fish#choice

October 5, S. B., and 2021. (2021, October 5). The #1 Best Fish to Eat to Reduce Inflammation, Says Science. Eat This Not That. Https: //www.eatthis.com/best-fish-to- reduce-inflammation/

Omega-3 Fatty Acids | Cleveland Clinicup (2019). Cleveland Clinicup https:

//my.clevelandclinicuporg/health/articles/17290-omega-3-fatty-acids

Pahwa, R., and Jialal, I. (2019, June 4). Chronic Inflammation. NIH.gov; statpearls Publishing. Https: //www.ncbi.nlm.nih.gov/books/NBK493173/

Pharm, J. (2020, June 23). Are Eggs Anti-Inflammatory? Medicinenet; medicinenet. Https: //www.medicinenet.com/are_eggs_anti-inflammatory/article.htm

Pineapple Juice: Are There Health Benefits? (2020, September). Webmd. Https:

//www.webmd.com/diet/pineapple-juice-health-benefits

Prebiotics - an overview | sciencedirect Topics. (2017). Www.sciencedirect.com. Https: //www.sciencedirect.com/topics/agricultural-and-biological-sciences/prebiotics6. https://www.ncbi.nlm.nih.gov/pmc/articles/PMC5476783/

https://www.ncbi.nlm.nih.gov/pubmed/26526061

https://www.ncbi.nlm.nih.gov/pubmed/22176839

https://www.ncbi.nlm.nih.gov/pmc/articles/PMC5932180/

https://www.ncbi.nlm.nih.gov/pmc/articles/PMC2839879/

https://www.ncbi.nlm.nih.gov/pubmed/19295480

https://www.mdmag.com/medical-news/amy-tyberg-md-gerd-as-an-inflammatory-disease

https://www.arthritis.org/health-wellness/healthy-living/nutrition/anti-inflammatory/anti-inflammatory-diet

https://www.ncbi.nlm.nih.gov/pubmed/24925270

https://www.ncbi.nlm.nih.gov/pubmed/24224694

https://www.ncbi.nlm.nih.gov/pubmed/26383493

https://www.hindawi.com/journals/jnme/2012/539426/

https://www.ncbi.nlm.nih.gov/pubmed/24552752

https://pubs.acs.org/doi/abs/10.1021/pr4008199

https://www.ahajournals.org/doi/10.1161/JAHA.118.011367

Dear readers,

As we conclude this book on the anti-inflammatory diet, we want to express our sincere appreciation for joining us on this enlightening journey. Thank you for your dedication and commitment to improving your health.

Before we part ways, we have some exciting bonuses in store for all of you. By scanning the QR code, you will have the opportunity to win an incredible prize to help you transform your life. Additionally, as a token of our gratitude, you will have access to an exclusive discount on a personalized meal plan, specifically created for you.

Do not miss out on these incredible opportunities to enhance your anti-inflammatory lifestyle. Scan the QR code now to unlock your bonuses and embark on a path to improved well-being

Here, you have the opportunity to make a difference. Don't just be a reader; become a collaborator with **THE FAN CLUB KITCHEN** to create even better books. Our cookbooks are uniquely crafted thanks to our readers themselves.

Unlock your potential and go beyond the role of a passive reader. Take a proactive step towards shaping the future of our culinary journeys. By completing the dedicated questionnaire, you will actively contribute to the creation of extraordinary books that cater to your needs and desires.

Your voice matters. Together, let's redefine the world of cooking literature. Join us in this empowering endeavor, and together, we will continue to produce exceptional works that inspire and delight.

Don't miss this opportunity to leave your mark. Be a part of something truly remarkable. Start now by sharing your invaluable insights and let us create the best cookbooks imaginably, fueled by the collective wisdom of our remarkable readers like you.

Made in the USA
Middletown, DE
08 July 2023

34730257R00077